LANDSCAPES IN MY MIND

LANDSCAPES IN MY MIND

THE ORIGINS AND STRUCTURE OF THE SUBJECTIVE EXPERIENCE

Vincenzo R. Sanguineti, M.D.

PSYCHOSOCIAL PRESS
MADISON   CONNECTICUT

Library of Congress Cataloging-in-Publication Data

Sanguineti, Vincenzo R.
  Landscapes in my mind : the origins and structure of the subjective experience / Vincenzo R. Sanguineti.
      p.   cm.
  Includes bibliographical references and indexes.
  ISBN 1–887841–25–3
    1. Subjectivity.   I. Title.
  BF697S2394   1999
  155.2—dc21   99–36302
                                                         CIP

Manufactured in the United States of America

Contents

Introduction ix

CHAPTER ONE
The Subjective Experience: A Brief Review 1
Subjectivity: A Definition 1
Subjectivity and Mental Research 6
Conclusions 27

CHAPTER TWO
Two Mentalistic Portraits 31
The Book and Its Content 31
The Author: A Vastly Condensed Version 43
Conclusions 49

CHAPTER THREE
Workings of the Mind: Consciousness and the
Unconscious 53
A Personal Vignette: "Finding the Road" 53
An Objective Example: "The Silicon Pretender" 61
Conclusions 67

CHAPTER FOUR
The Unfolding of Life: The Genetic
Endowment 69
A Personal Vignette: "Meet the Gazelle" 69
*An Objective Example: "Preaching to the
Creatures"* 76
Conclusions 85

CHAPTER FIVE
The Evolutionary Archetypes: Values and
Needs 87
A Personal Vignette: "Making a Fire" 87
An Objective Example: "The Master" 96
Conclusions 100

CHAPTER SIX

One of the Line: Values and Needs   103
A Personal Vignette: "The Shell, the Urn"   103
An Objective Example: "What My Father Told Me"   112
Conclusions   115

CHAPTER SEVEN

Affective Connectedness: The Qualia Web   117
Affectivity   118
Interactive Reality   121
Intentionality   124
A Personal Vignette: "I Lost My Hat"   126
An Objective Example: "The Universe of Objects"   129
Conclusions   132

CHAPTER EIGHT

Talking to the Stars: The Quanta Web   135
Personal Reflections   135
An Objective Example: "The Undiscovered Element"   143
Conclusions   146

CHAPTER NINE

Putting It All Together   149
A Personal Vignette: "The Kitchen Counter"   149
An Objective Example: "Psyche and Eros"   153
Conclusions   158

CHAPTER TEN

Some Closing Reflections   159

References   167

Name Index   171

Subject Index   173

This world isn't old enough for anyone to be removed by more than six
degrees of blood from anyone else.
Gods included. (The goddess Siveni
and Diane Duane, among others)

Introduction

The subjective mind is a mystery
within a mystery. (V. Sanguineti)

J was slouched in the seat, head downcast, stooped shoulders, lifeless. I asked her, "What is this sadness about?"

Her left hand went to her hair, adjusted a curl behind her left ear.[1]

He sat straight against the tall back of the leather armchair, comfortably filling its space. His face was in full profile. In my mind's eye I saw the shimmering hologram of a black-and-white feather, an eagle's feather, hanging on his left shoulder from a tress of black hair. I knew him well; I had met him for the first time when she lay in the intensive care unit, comatose from an overdose. He had come, when called, to slow her heart from beating madly 200 times each minute to a safe rhythm of 84 beats.

His name was K, a full-blooded Comanche warrior as they used to be when the prairie was nothing but prairie; the keeper of the body's mysteries, the pain controller. Now he sat there and told me not to hurt her and spoke of winds and eagles—the feather dangling in my mind, behind his ear—and of the difficult task of

---

[1]The author wants readers to *immediately* experience the perplexing, uncertain, at times confusing state that accompanies all explorations into the realm of the subjective.

caring for the sick ones, particularly her; and of his duty that no one should die.

"No one will die," I said. His left hand rose to adjust the feather.

She turned her chair to face me, straight and tall and said in her strong, categorical voice: "Listen to your tape, of the session you had with J on October 13th 2 years ago. It was 5:26 by your clock. J had spoken in a soft voice and the heavy rain lashing against the windows had covered her words. You asked her to repeat what she had told you, louder this time. J repeated: 'I do not want to disappear, to die,' and you responded, 'You will not die; you will take the others with you and be complete.' "

"Do not try to tell us that no one will die," she concluded.

I recognized her too: T, the keeper of memories. Like the writer Jorge Luis Borges' fictional Funes the Memorius (1964a) who "knew by heart the forms of the southern clouds at dawn on the 30th of April, 1882" (p. 63), all that had been and had been told was present in her, unchanged. "Do not try to tell us that no one will die," T then added.

"You certainly remember my explanations," I answered. "I never spoke of death."

"I do remember quite well, as you have come to find out," she replied, distant and neutral in the tone of her voice. "If we give up who we are then we are not at all. You too would cease to exist if you lost your identity. Some of us are very scared," she added. She then adjusted the curl behind her left ear.[2]

---

[2]It is common in a multiple personality system for a specific movement or change in body posture to trigger or signal the transition between alter states.

I met her eyes, shining with animated light; she appeared almost weightless, more slim that usual. To my mind her voice carried unsung songs. I knew her quite well and felt the usual tinge of pleasure that accompanied all her visits. She had spoken at length of enchanted woods in a younger world and in another land. She lived in those woods, in a protected castle. Elfinlike magic would keep a perennial wall of mirth and unbound Nature to surround and seal her realm. All her alters knew how she could reach my mind, and so they used to "send" her, to prove me wrong, to bend me in the illusion of her existence, to negotiate the survival of them all, lest I lose her too, in the process of integration. (Integration is the final step in the therapy of these cases, through which the distinctiveness of multiplicity is undone, and the splintered many become one consolidated self.)

Within less than one hour I had been exposed to three alternate worlds, three alternate selves. Each one was alive as the carrier of them all, the original depressed woman who now sat again in front of me. She sat there, folded unto her own self, dejected, without memory of what and whom had transpired, aware only—by looking at the clock—of having once more experienced an episode of time loss.

This *one* human mind contained within her a set of complex independent landscapes. A score of selves subjectively experienced their own existence as absolutely real and independent from each other. They all competed for one body, and for the right to live.

The case represented one of many experiences of a similar nature encountered during years spent quietly observing the subjective architecture of human minds unfolding through the process of psychotherapy. Possibly, the exploration of a multiple personality reveals to its extreme the role of the subjective experience in the configuration of reality and the simultaneity and intricate interplay of different psychic organizations, each with its own distinctive structure in space and time. This book can be viewed as an attempt to deal with the elusive and apparently ever changing quality of such subjective experiences, a quality that has always put subjectivity at odds with traditional mental science. Out of this conflict subjectivity has been largely expressed through art and literature and has been avoided as a topic by scientists of the mind. So, although within the realm of consciousness the subjective element forms the most intimate and complete representation of our true self, it is probably accurate to say that we have not advanced much from the position of William James (1890/1950). Possibly we have regressed, in that his fringe experience concept has been devalued or ignored.[3] In my opinion several reasons justify this reticence. First, this material is difficult to manipulate and to subject to statistical evaluation. A more compelling reason may involve the individual's reluctance to engage in self-disclosure. Unmodified subjective material is difficult to produce, because it implies and requires a significant degree of self-exposure and a candid delivery of its meaning. By having our most precious and personal self—our true nature—really known to others we may become defenseless against devaluation. D. Galin

---

[3]James recognized two parts to awareness: the nucleus (or the definite) and the fringe (or the vague), and suggested that these two parts contain qualitatively different sets of data. Fringe experiences constitute all the interrelated data that eventually give meaning and context to the nucleus. Among these experiences he mentioned feelings of rightness, familiarity, knowing, and relatedness.

(1995), in discussing the reluctance to talk about the subjective experience that he observed at a symposium on consciousness, suggested as a cause that "the topic seems to provoke both extreme skittishness and extreme fascination. Research on subjective experience is like sex; everybody is terribly interested in it but does not want to be caught in public doing it" (p. 4). I certainly felt rather naked and undefended while I wrote and revised those subjective experiences of mine that are described as vignettes throughout the book. And yet the subjective is so central to mental operations that it cannot be circumvented without critically undermining any research in the field. When viewed from such a perspective, this book constitutes a renewed effort, in the present literature on mental science, to report subjective experiences in their entirety and in terms suitable for objective evaluation, and to deal with the topic of subjectivity in an organized way. In doing so it offers robust data to verify two cardinal claims. (These claims have been theoretically formulated by scores of researchers, but they generally lack endorsement from any set of data presented in a systematic way.)

1. The mental self develops out of a vast set of mentalistic programs, some of which can be traced to the prehuman phases of cerebral (and mental) development (this process parallels the development of the physical self).

2. The entire information in a human mind appears to be operative as a gestalt, *in its entirety,* during most, if not all, mental operations. Such mode of function strongly suggests that the brain–mind complex operates also in ways consistent with the laws of quantum physics, and not only at the classical Newtonian level. This level indicates the aspect of reality that is based on Newton's

laws of universal gravitation. In such reality accurately quantified forces predictably direct the interaction of all elementary units that constitute the basis of all processes. Newtonian mechanics, with its set of forces and laws, became the only and true scientific paradigm. All phenomena in nature can be precisely explained in terms of a few basic laws; the entire reality can be viewed as a very complex but mechanical system operating in a highly predictable, linear, computational way. Time is an external and unidirectional factor and deterministic laws direct all natural events. The cause-and-effect principle rules the universe, including the human mind.

Quantum theory, on the contrary, posits a fundamental indeterminism at the very basis of nature that does not allow for individual events to be predicted or calculated in a precise way. The most significant aspects of quantum physics will be described in greater detail later on in the text.

The foundations of the book consist of four supporting points, and specific vignettes are used to illustrate these points.

1. *All conscious thoughts are the emergent outcome of processes that are largely not conscious.* The intuitive property of the mind is a major representation of this concept. The importance of intuition in organizing the "invisible sea" that supports and colors all our subjective experiences—and the vastness of such a sea—is therefore discussed first, to introduce the thesis that consciousness is the condensed expression of multidetermined mental operations that may involve our global knowledge.

2. *The data that contribute to or form our global knowledge have different origins.* The first category of these data is inherited in nature. This library of inherited

knowledge can be further subdivided into three orders, each one representing an emergent outcome from the preceding one.

(a)   The first order includes information about evolutionary adaptations that preceded the differentiation of our genus Homo from its predecessors. We share these data—mentalistic as well as physical—with other species. The experience of territoriality and the related adaptive signals that modulate competitiveness are introduced to the reader very early, as instances of this type of data, as well as themes of emotional "recognition," of exploratory curiosity, of empathy for psychophysical distress that appear to cross the divide between species.

(b)   A second order of inherited knowledge contains data about the very early roots of the human mind: primal human evolution and the emergence of specific values and needs.

(c)   A third order of genetic knowledge contains information about a narrower evolutionary sequence, that I have labeled the "ancestors' line." This line represents inherited favorite templates and data about a specific cultural niche and social structure, and related specific elaborations of primitive values and needs.

The second category of data that contribute to our global knowledge represents all that we experience during our individual lifetime. These last data are processed through the data from the first category, and constantly reclassify and reorganize them. This interactive process is responsible for the exquisitely subjective and ever changing characteristics of our minds.

3. *A shared attribute of this myriad of data is their being weighted with affective elements or qualia.* *Affectivity* is used in this context as a technical term that defines a family of states and events for which a "feeling" characteristic represents a primary attribute of each state. Affectivity and affective resonance constitute a communal pathway to the workings of the mind.

4. *All this information is continuously available and potentially active during any and all mental activity.* The vastness of the simultaneous activation of the entire mental gestalt is the major theme and challenge of the book. The characteristics of such activation have interesting similarities to some of the characteristics of the world of quantum mechanics—a very fashionable theme in the mental sciences—that may offer some scientific corroboration to my subjective description of my inner mental world.

The book is also dedicated to all researchers and students of the mind, irrespective of creed, for having enriched my understanding; and it seeks their critical interest. It represents my personal contribution to all those among us who experience and cherish their ultimate subjective essence, who may be curious as to the complex contents of its structures, and touched by the marvel and polymorphism of all mental landscapes. Subjectivity may indeed prove to be the ultimate and most *universal* of all human frontiers.

CHAPTER ONE

The Subjective Experience: A Brief Review

> There is no human experience, nor would experience be possible at all, without the intervention of a subjective aptitude. What is this subjective aptitude? Ultimately it consists of an innate psychic structure which allows men to have experiences of this kind.
> (C. G. Jung, 1953/1977, p. 190)

Subjectivity: A Definition

An initial difficulty in organizing a systematic presentation of the topic of subjectivity resides in its definition. Perhaps not surprisingly, I am still struggling with the enunciation of an orthodox, concise set of words that would semantically describe the entire concept. Such difficulty may be related to the presence and prevalence of the innumerable precognitive and largely wordless, nonconscious aspects of the subjective architecture. Still, I will at least try, with the help of a thought experiment, to draw a broad differentiation between the subjective and the nonsubjective aspects of brain–mind function. In so doing I will clarify the scope and the limitations of my work.

1

I lie in the reclining surgical chair. The mask of the controlled image releaser (CIR) is set with a tight seal over my face and I stare into the dense gray fog that fills the mask and my entire visual field. At carefully calculated intervals the image of a ripe, red apple flashes rapidly in the center of the field. Nearby, the neurosurgical team observes on a monitor the patterns of graded colored concentrations painted on my brain by the precisely titrated sequential infusions of radio-labeled chemicals. The apple appearances illuminate a bright and stable web of interconnected pathways, easily recognizable among the variegated and unstable permutations of diffuse colors that reflect the distribution of each wave of radioisotopes. The composite computerized image of the web becomes clearer with each successive stimulus and its definition increases (as a shallow reef would do by breaking the progression of the waves to the shore). This tridimensional web traces the "apple-perceiving" phenomena from the retinal cells of my eyes to the "recognition" centers in my occipital lobe. It also includes the predicted branch to the labeling site in my brain.

In a nearby surgical recliner you undergo the same procedure: you too are repeatedly presented with an identical image of a red apple as precisely positioned as mine is. Your neurosurgical team observes in the monitor the same web of stimulus perception. The computer now superimposes our two webs on the upper half of each screen, while continuously upgrading the images as more information keeps adding with each new exposure. Predictably, the two images are remarkably similar and allow for a very gratifying level of matching. Only minor blurs, well within acceptable variance, interrupt the clarity of the juxtaposed design.

The neurosurgical transplant team, satisfied with the high compatibility of the two images, applies the probes of the electrochemical transplanter (ECT) to a preformed window in my skull. With astounding precision the probes gradually recognize and dissect the apple-web along its electrochemical boundaries with the rest of my neural tissue. Microchemical and electrical markers are left at each synaptic stump site for future recognition. As the process unfolds the dissected part of the web is instantly surrounded by the feeding broth that keeps it alive and protects its architecture in space from any disruptive mechanical stress.

At the nearby recliner your apple-web is similarly dissected away. Once the dissections are completed the broth-filled containers slide on their tracks from one recliner to the other. The ECT mode is reversed, and each transplanter begins the delicate and precise process of identifying each marker and rebuilding the electrochemical bonds between the transplanted parts and the rest of the organ. Minute adjustments (the blurs in the juxtaposed pictures) are gently smoothed over through the plasticity of the surrounding tissues.

The two-way transplant is now complete. We both recognize with absolute ease the red apple that flashes inside our CIR.

What you and I have been subjected to is a transplant of the "stimulus perception and recognition" neural circuitry in our brain. This circuitry transmits the attributes of external reality deep into the brain, and it does so in a computational and highly predictable way. The process is a significant aspect of consciousness as well as nonconscious automatic monitoring of external reality. *But it is not subjectivity.*

Whenever the dense fog inside the CIR is pierced by the image of a red apple another major set of events is put in motion. During each single experience the attributes of the external object are processed through and modified by the composite attributes of my internal reality of "Apple." These internal attributes—conglomerates of singular experiences—span the period from this most recent one in a surgical chair to early experiences of childhood in war-ravaged Northern Italy, when even the child recognized food as a very scarce commodity and survival as very uncertain. They may even link to primal information on food experiences and related values acquired at the origin of the species or of Life itself. This set of mine is profoundly different from the analogous process that becomes activated in your brain whenever you see the red apple emerging in the fog of your CIR.

This is what constitutes subjectivity: the processing of all that we experience through our own personal *inclinations*. These inclinations represent the result of the interplay of inherited and acquired material. They infuse the algorithmic workings of the neural circuitry with our ever changing, always updated interpretation of the world that surrounds us, of our own selves, and of the interactive processes between the two systems.

Each perception is inexorably accompanied by a process of scrutiny and by the activation of memories, meanings, values, intentional states, and emotional correlates. All these activities involve the entire brain and require that distinct brain areas enter an interconnected and multifunctional mode. Such background is the crucial component that invests the brutish, replicable neural machinery with those unique attributes that differentiate each individual's final mental outcomes.

Mental functioning, including consciousness, is fundamentally the elaboration of the entirety of our subjective gestalts that cover our personal space-time and may even span other dimensions, such as the prehuman and protohuman. I suggest that this invisible sea of data (experiential, affective, intentional, value-laden) is potentially present at all times for all mental operations. This concept of global cerebral functioning has become a subject of exploration in neuroscience, through the application of the nonlinear dynamics branch of mathematics. Mathematician A. C. Scott (1995) explains how "the term *nonlinear* is defined in the context of the relationship between cause and effect" (p. 189). In linear mathematics it is relatively simple to understand how a system works. Scott goes on to say: "Linear systems are much easier to analyze than nonlinear systems, since a complex cause can be expressed as a convenient sum of simple components, and the combined effect is the sum of the effects from each component of the total cause. For this reason linear systems have been favored by physical scientists, especially during the current century" (p. 189).

In the nonlinear realm, however, "the effect from the sum of two causes is not equal to the sum of the individual effects. The whole is not equal to the sum of its parts" (p. 189). Scott also advocates that "nonlinear phenomena are by far the more natural and commonplace in biology" (p. 4). As examples of such nonlinear phenomena he uses a flock of geese, a poem about a past experience, a tornado developing out of a storm. He then continues: "It should be no surprise that consciousness, a biological reality even to children, is yet another instance of such nonlinear coherence. Consciousness *emerges*" (p. 5).

By the use of this science researchers from several disciplines (physics, neurophysiology, mathematics, neuroscience) are trying to understand the "collective dynamics of billions of interconnected neurons in the brain" (Glanz, 1997). As I will discuss in the following chapters, these global dynamics may involve a subneuronal, presynaptic level of phenomena alongside the more traditional neuronal plane.

The task of this book is to present sufficiently comprehensive data retrieved from my personal sea to support the sources and the vastness of my subjective world.

Subjectivity and Mental Research

Despite the centrality of subjectivity to the workings of the mind, a search of the literature on this function demonstrates scarcity of information and organized knowledge as to what constitutes the subjective experience. For instance, in the report from the Tucson debates on consciousness the term *subjective experience* was cited three times. Of these, only a paper by Galin (1996) that surveyed past theories and the commonly used terminology dealt with the topic to any extent. "Subjectivity" was mentioned in a brief overview by Harman (1996) that proposes specific epistemological criteria. In order to maintain scientific objectivity, researchers try to explore the minds of others, or to construct abstract metaphors of what a mind might be. I contend that the only mind that we may grasp is our own, because the subjective element is central both to the search and to the understanding (an extension of the Socratic "know thyself"). Common sense tells us so; we all instinctively know the difference between our self-perception and our perception of others. And yet we think that we cannot understand the mind unless we study those of others, *deprived of their own subjectivity.*

This book does not try to explain how mentalistic states arise or how the mind functions. I will, however, present here some of my concerns about the current techniques in mental research. I affirm that when a science of the mind is unwilling to accept the centrality of subjectivity and its major role in delivering information about mental events, then that science is dead in the water. Mental states cannot be grasped, and therefore understood, without being observed and communicated from an internal perspective and experience. It is quite understandable that such proposition may be—to paraphrase the philosopher John Searle (1992)—terrifying to any scientist: the subjective search appears to preclude objective verification. (Searle says, "The deepest reason for the fear of consciousness is that consciousness has the essentially terrifying feature of subjectivity" [p. 55].) But it seems to me that we have to live with the risk, if we want to begin collecting valid information about mental operations, particularly the ones that constitute major functions: consciousness, nonconscious processes, emotions, intentionality, values, needs, experiential learning, and subjective adaptation.

A further consideration: Objective studies of mental phenomena "observe" a very incomplete translation, truncated by the inevitably reductionistic study design, of a subjective event (like the perception and the response to a specific stimulus). The chain of events linking perception of the stimulus to response is not understood. The subject is usually unaware with regard to the full range and magnitude of the steps involved in the process (an example of the wondrous complexity contained in apparently simple mentalistic processes is presented in chapter 7). Yet the subject is asked to report the perception–response package either through a preprogrammed set of brief descriptions or by performing a specific, simplified action-response. Such report is then taken as representing the entire chain process. The objective observer may try to use rigid classical parameters in order to consistently replicate the

same chain of events, but would still be unable to avoid
the centrality of the subjective experience from pervad-
ing even these limited and rather artificial psychic activities. The objective observer can only fabricate a
pseudoreality by pretending to exclude the wondrous
symphony of Sherrington's (1951) *enchanted loom*[1] that
keeps dancing through the subject's mind. Indeed, the
elaboration of "mentalistic" data may be as affected
by the subjective experience in objective studies as in
subjective ones, albeit through different processes.

We are increasingly aware that the very act of observation affects the results not only in the quantum realm
but also in the realm of classical reality. In all objective
studies *both* investigator and subject bring the weight
of their mental states (unconscious processing, values,
needs, intentionality networks, emotional inclinations)
to bear on the conscious understanding of the data and
of the conclusions reached from the investigations. We
now have *two* sets of mental states to reckon with.

This "observer effect" may indeed assume even
greater relevance when the subjects of the study are minute components of very complex mentalistic events,
unattached flickers in the enchanted loom, as in the
case of an isolated behavioral response.

The replicability argument (that for a scientific
study to be considered valid it is necessary that it could
be replicable in its design as well as its results) is therefore a specious one: these "objective" studies share the
bias of the design itself, in addition to internal causes for

---

[1] "The brain is waking and with it the mind is returning. It is as if the
Milky Way entered upon some cosmic dance. Swiftly the head mass becomes
*an enchanted loom where millions of flashing shuttles weave a dissolving pattern,
always a meaningful pattern though never an abiding one; a shifting of subpatterns*"
(as reported in Scott 1995, p. 75; emphasis added).

misinterpretation. A widespread example of artificial, misleading design is offered by the traditional "intelligence" tests, where thought is confused with reasoning, and a function labeled "intelligence" is assessed while being neither understood nor properly defined. Intuition could be considered a dominant component of "intelligence," and yet its probable key mental mechanism—analogic thinking and "creativity," i.e., divergent thinking (Kogan, [1980], as reported in Gelernter, [1994])—cannot be captured by the standard test designs that are centered on convergent thinking and on manifest, highly focused consciousness states. Another interesting instance of design inadequacy may be a curious phenomenon linked with the perception of ambiguous mental states. Both the Necker cube and the Schroder stairs (Figure 1.1) are ambiguous figures; each of these figures can be perceived in two different, alternating ways. Various hypotheses have been advanced to explain the phenomenon: gestalt psychology accounts for it as if each perception were due to a different neural assembly that, however, could not be sustained because of habituation and of competitive recruiting from the other assembly.

You may experiment with an interesting twist to this test. Concentrate on the cube in Figure 1.1 till it "jumps" to the second configuration. You may then notice at the periphery of your vision that the stairs have "jumped" too. If you keep rearranging your perception of the cube you may also notice that the two drawings appear to be locked in a specific configuration: in my case if the cube's frontal face looks toward me and to my left, then the stairs will go up toward the left; if the cube's front face looks up and to my right, then the stairs will be suspended upside down. I have not found

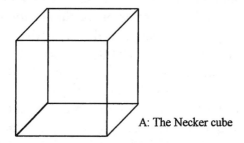

A: The Necker cube

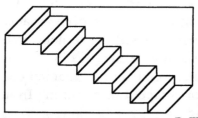

B: The Schroder stairs

Figure 1.1   The spatial organization of the ambiguous figure under observation affects the entire surrounding visual field and not only the more narrow area of direct observation. Consequently, when the observer triggers a change in the spatial orientation of one figure, such change provokes a reorganization of the entire visual field. Any aspect of reality present in the field and carrying some ambiguity in its configuration will therefore be subject to corresponding simultaneous changes in its spatial organization.

this peculiarity described anywhere in the literature about ambiguous figures, possibly because the experiment design does not consider what happens to perception beyond the boundaries of the stimulus: these figures are usually presented one at a time. When the "ambiguous image" problem is looked at in this light it may imply different mechanisms from the ones traditionally called upon for an explanation; one may speculate that once the brain is set on a particular spatial orientation it tends to process different realities in the same way. It could rather successfully do that, whenever these realities are sufficiently ambiguous to allow for such function (the topic will be discussed again in chapter 7).

The richness of data from subjective studies is vastly superior to the reduced and simplified data available to and from objective investigation. As a general rule, the data from objective investigations are limited to the cognitive, sequential, "communicable," worded category. All the nameless emotional states and gestaltic structures contributing to all mental operations could not be captured and are indeed actively avoided by most objective studies, that often also demand the support of classical algorithmic procedures. The introduction of subjective data would certainly complicate the understanding of mentalistic phenomena, but is nevertheless essential to such understanding. Without it all studies would be limited to the phenomenological shell empty of individuality, and to reductive functionalism.

Allow me to guide you through another exercise in illustrating what I allude to when I mention the subjective experience and its role in the perception of reality. We may walk into the Picasso room at the Museo Nacional Centro de Arte Reina Sofia in Madrid or enter St.

Peter's Basilica in Rome and turn right toward the first absid. In the first case we are faced with the Guernica by Picasso. In the second case we will be looking at the Pietá by Michelangelo. These two artistic expressions are quite different from each other. Still, when facing them we may perceive a stirring, inside. We may feel a vague connection and wonderment. These masterpieces move us. I stand there, open to some arcane message on the canvas or in the marble. Then someone nearby informs me that I am looking at a replica; the original has been relocated, and can be viewed at another site nearby.

At this precise point the observable reality in front of me loses "depth" (or something); the "movement" in me flattens out, vanishes. I may thoroughly admire the mastery of the copy maker, but the reproduction lacks something tangible. It misses this tangible, indescribable entity to such an extent that, without hesitation, I move to the site of the original. I then reexperience the "something" that the copy could not convey.

I am not really sure what this something is. It may be wonderment at the creative process and at the passion of Picasso or Michelangelo. It may be echoes from their subjective working in seeking an emergent symbol, on the canvas and in the marble, for their inner encompassing gestalt: a faint recognition of and empathy for the message-theme behind their creation. In the world of classical reality, of objective consciousness, clearly we both looked at the apple and its "identical twin," when we looked at the original and at the copy. Still, they are quite different.

I propose that the difference resides in the field of subjectivity, perhaps in the areas of meanings and value systems. The subjective field interacts with reality (see interactive reality in chapter 7) and colors it with (personalized) meaning and value. And I *know* that the copy maker did not experience, during the task, anything resembling what was in the mind of Picasso or Michelangelo. The two "apples" may look identical to the objective observer, but as an internal experience they are incommensurably diverse. They are, to all intents, different realities.

I also propose that all strictly objective approaches to the investigation of true consciousness fail to take into account the permutable, immense, ongoing connectedness of the (human) brain. Scott (1995, p. 20) reports the immensity of the number of possible mental systems, supported by 10 billion neurons (10^{10}) each of which has a conservative number of synaptic inputs = 10^4, for a total conservative number of mental states of $10^{10^{17}}$. This conservative number is the *immense* number of physicist Elsasser (1969) who labels as immense numbers all finite numbers greater than 10^{110}, which roughly represents the atomic mass of the universe multiplied by its age measured in picoseconds, multiplied by itself 10,000 trillion times. A very large number indeed.

And yet this number may represent a very partial view of the real complexity of an operational brain. A very lively sector of neuroscience research (that will be outlined later in the text) suggests that the synaptic architecture is only the final phase of an organization that begins in the subneuronal realm of quantum states operating along the microtubular structure of the neuron and of the glial cells. The value reported above by Scott would then simply pale in comparison with the number of possible permutations from the combination of these two dynamic systems, the presynaptic (or subneuronal) and the synaptic.

It follows that all research on the mind based on the stimulus–response paradigm could be compared to research on an entire culture based on the repeated observation of one isolated individual answering selected and simple mathematical questions. Clearly, this objective technique is too reductionistic. For a true understanding of the mind we need to reconsider the approach to be used. We need to tap into the subjective description of mental activity as the only currently available source for the collection of adequate data supported by a sufficient background awareness (self-awareness) of the true extent and composition of the mental phenomenon under study. The future of the controversial science of subjectivity rests, at least for now, on our willingness to accept the subject as being also the observer and that some degree of unreplicability is a cardinal aspect of humanhood and selfhood.

Asimov (1991a) fictionally recalled that "grimly, Man had instinctively sought to circumvent the prison bars of ordinary speech. Semantics, symbolic logic, psychoanalysis—they had all been devices whereby speech could either be refined or bypassed" (p. 118). The major contributions to a true breakthrough in the understanding of human mental functioning came from the various forms of analysis of the psyche, that used the subjective experience as the main source of information, and carefully tried to avoid contamination from the objective observer (as in countertransference phenomena).[2]

---

[2]Countertransference is a specific process first described in the psychoanalytic literature, by which the therapist who is presented with mental material by the subject vests such material with his or her own personal meanings. Therefore the subjective material is redesigned along the therapist's value system and becomes contaminated by such *transfer* which results into a new landscape being built that reflects both sources (both minds).

Once such information is actively solicited and accepted as a valid representation of what really happens, we would then be able to apply our intuition and to search for tools, techniques, and designs that would adequately reflect the reality of the task. Simplification and reductionism do necessarily corrupt the method used and foster results that represent less the true reality under study than hypothetical constructs based on only one isolated attribute of reality.

I will occasionally refer to some models of mental function that are particularly appealing to me: from the theories of quantum consciousness as supported by neurophysiologist John Eccles (1993), mathematician Roger Penrose (1994), and physicist John Herbert (1993) among others, to the neural Darwinism model of neuroscientist Gerald Edelman (1992) or the gestaltic view of neuropharmacologist Susan Greenfield (1995), and the affect-based system of computer scientist David Gelernter (1994). The design that will emerge out of these pages (summarized in Figure 1.2) has a significant resemblance to the hierarchical system described by Scott. Therefore, I will now submit a brief outline of these schemes and theories. However, all these systems represent hypothetical, speculative paradigms. What is not hypothetical or speculative, in this book, is the set of descriptions of my own mental activity: these descriptions receive a quite robust documentation by means of a series of data that I retrieved from within myself at a significant personal cost and change. Because of my experience I fully agree with the speculation raised by Harman (1996) who advises that "the researcher must be willing to risk being profoundly changed through the process of exploration" (p. 748).

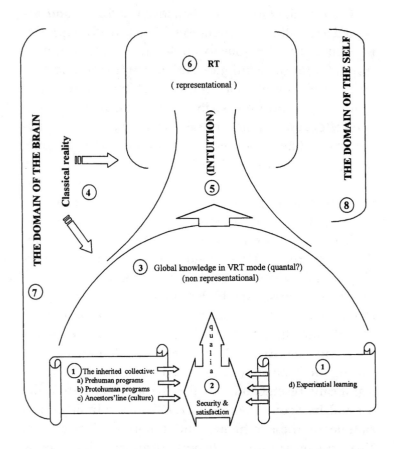

Figure 1.2 A map of my mind (1) adaptational data developed during evolution and common to many species (a), to the entire hominid line (b) and to socio-cultural organizations (c) constantly interact with data from the individual's experiential learning (d). These data are processed for basic survival value (2) and are in this way categorized and weighted with qualia (affective loading): the data constitute our global knowledge (3) and are available in a global way (nonlinear dynamics?) at a nonrepresentational state (very rapid thinking [VRT]; quantum states?). Under demand from classical reality (4) these states collapse into representational constructs or RT (6); the transformation may be perceived as *intuition* (5). These last constructs allow for internal as well as external communication and interaction and may involve discrete neuronal networks. Both sets of function (VRT and RT) are within the domain of the brain (7): the self (the brain's interactive "persona") is limited to the RT domain (8)? (See text for clarification on specific terms.)

Often these data are further supported by a strong intuitive component that suggests an internal "proof of truth," a t-test of sorts (self-evidently such a state does not imply an objective, Platonic truth; it simply conveys a strong message of complete *consistency* among all my internal hierarchies of data).

Theories of Quantum Consciousness[3]

Several experts have tried to translate and summarize quantum science and its relationship to mind into concepts accessible to nonphysicists. According to Nick Herbert (1993), three features of the quantum world appear to be most important for models of the mind.

The first feature that characterizes the quantum world and differentiates it from the Newtonian dimension is *quantum randomness* (or *quantum indeterminancy*). When an atom is observed under specific conditions the atom will appear as a particle, and the particular attributes chosen for the observation will show definite values. At a second observation the atom would still look like a particle. In the observed state it appears to conform with Newtonian laws and expectations. But if the observer tries to conceptualize the atom as a particle in between observations, he or she will not be able to accurately predict the results of the second observation. The atom seems now to escape the Newtonian laws being used to predict its behavior.

[If the observer] describes the unobserved atom in the peculiar quantum manner as a *wave of possibilities*, he gets

---

[3]Readers who may not want to be bothered with scientific theories, at least for the time being, can skip directly to page 26 and return to these scientific models when needed.

the right result every time for the second observation. What does it mean to represent an atom as a wave of possibilities? Instead of being located in one place like an ordinary object, the unobserved atom is represented, by a mathematical formula called the atom's wave function, as being in many possible places at the same time. (Herbert, 1993, p. 144)

The process of observation appears to transform the randomness implicit in the wave state into a particle state with definite attributes. This phenomenon is called collapse of the wave function, or quantum leap. Implicit in the model is the potential for a variety of different outcomes from a single situation or from identical situations. Furthermore, according to Herbert, the feature may offer some substance to the suggestion that the factors affecting the collapse may not lie in the physical world: "the ultimate cause of material phenomena is not material at all but stems from an essentially mental realm" (p. 174).

The second feature is *quantum thinglessness.* In Newtonian reality every object has specific attributes, irrespective of the presence or absence of an observer, that can always be precisely measured (at least in theory) in isolation from each other. In the quantum world, on the contrary, each single attribute appears to be inextricably linked to one or more different attributes. The act of measuring a specific attribute consequently excludes the separate measurement of those other attributes that are linked to the one under study. Therefore, the reality being observed appears to be defined by the observer's choice of a specific aspect or attribute at the exclusion of others. This mode of observation is reminiscent of the aspectual characteristic of intentional states described by Searle (1992) and reported in the next chapter.

Furthermore, the observed reality is then further defined by the quantum randomness principle, that will determine the particular expression, in the dimension of classical reality, for the attribute that is being observed. Herbert states that "a quantum mind faces the same measurement problem when it desires to manifest some aspect of reality. First it must form (or find) a context for its contemplated actions. Then, within this context, it selects a particular value for the quantum attribute evoked by that context" (p. 179).

The third feature is possibly the most intriguing feature of quantum wave systems. It consists of the fact that once such systems have interacted they become so entangled that each future change, or action, on one system will "instantly and without mediation" (Herbert, 1993, p. 149) cause correlated changes in the second system. The two systems become a single entity, irrespective of their spatial relationship to each other.

> If one takes seriously this feature, called *quantum insepa-rability* (emphasis added), then all objects that have once interacted are in some sense still connected. Since this nonlocal connection does not actually stretch across space, it does not diminish with distance . . . likewise it takes up no time. A nonlocal connection leaps . . . faster than light. (p. 180)

As I will discuss again, this quantum inseparability represents an appealing possible explanation for the unity of our mental experiences.

The search for sites and models of quantum activity in the brain has been rather active. Neurophysiologist John Eccles (1993) identifies the site for quantum action at the presynaptic vesicular grid, where probability fields—possibly activated by "mental concentration involved in intention or planned thinking" (p. 189)—control the release of a transmitter vesicle. Mathematician Roger Penrose (1994) locates the site for quantum events in the cytoskeleton of the neurons and more specifically in its microtubular structures where, he asserts, one could find conditions sufficient to support in vivo quantum events. Quantum states may represent only one aspect, or level, in a hierarchical system where several diverse sets of nonlinear laws forge level-specific emergent outcomes.

Neural Darwinism or Theory of Neuronal Group Selection (TNGS)

The TNGS expounded by neuroscientist and Nobelian Gerald Edelman (1992) rests on the premise that genetic codes provide the blueprint for the broad development of the nervous system, by designing and activating the extremely complex processes of cell migration and reorganization that characterize the early phases of its development. The theory itself is based on three tenets. The first tenet, or developmental selection, deals with the impact of the dynamics of epigenetic competitive development upon the ultimate organization of each specific brain for each specific species. Edelman concludes that:

> [T]his entire process is a selectional one, involving populations of neurons engaged in topobiological *competition*. A population of variant groups of neurons in a given brain region, comprising neural networks arising by processes of somatic selection, is known as a *primary repertoire*. The genetic code does not provide a specific wiring

diagram for this repertoire. Rather, it imposes a set of *constraints* on the selectional process. Even with such constraints, genetically identical individuals are unlikely to have identical wiring, for selection is epigenetic. (p. 83)

The second tenet assumes that synaptic function reinforces and selects, throught specific biochemical processes, distinct organizations of neurons while lack of function would weaken unused synaptic connections. "This mechanism . . . effectively 'carves out' a variety of functioning *circuits* (with strengthened synapses) from the anatomical network by selection. Such a set of variant functional circuits is called a *secondary repertoire*" (p. 85).

The third tenet illustrates how information is constantly recycled to allow for the recognition of incoming perceptions and for the reelaboration and ongoing categorization of all the data through progressively more complex neuronal systems that eventually produce consciousness.

> [This tenet] is concerned with how the selectional events described in the first two tenets act to connect psychology to physiology. It suggests how brain maps interact by a process called reentry. This is perhaps the most important of all the proposals of the theory, for it underlies how the brain areas that emerge in evolution coordinate with each other to yield new functions. (p. 85; see also Figure 4.1)

The Concentric Theory of Consciousness

Neuroscientist Susan Greenfield (1995) describes the functions of the (conscious) mind as based on gestalts, "*a highly variable aggregation of neurons that is temporarily recruited around a triggering epicenter''* (p. 112). In her theory a gestalt is therefore a neuronal assembly and consciousness is considered to be "an emergent property" (p. 161). Although Greenfield stays largely within the supranuclear, neuronal level of mental activity, she also considers the possible role of quantum mechanics in the functioning of the mind. She describes how algorithmic computation may not be "the most appropriate description of operations in the brain leading to consciousness" (p. 155) and speculates that the gestalts could be organized along the principles of the quantum world. In this sense her structural neuronal gestalts appear to be consonant with the functional experiences that I describe and with which they share many characteristics, including nonlocality and simultaneity.

Affect and Thought: High and Low Focus States

Gelernter (1994) envisions a spectrum of ways to think that depends on the level of mental focus active at that specific time. He considers a high, a middle, and a low range of mental focus. These ranges may change from moment to moment, depending on many factors as fatigue or stimulation, distractions, or subliminal inner physiological states.

The high focus range provides the ground for analytical, penetrating thinking. As Gelernter indicates, "almost all attempts to simulate thought on a computer have dealt exclusively with this narrow, high-focus band at the top of the spectrum" (p. 5). Very little research in artificial intelligence tried to reproduce the medium range of focus, and none dealt with the low range. In the medium focus range "thinking becomes less penetrating and more diffuse" (p. 5). Gelernter thinks that beginning with this shift in focus downwards the emotional content begins to prevail upon the logical, problem-solving mode in directing thought production. Finally he describes a low focus state: "the mental state that we might informally call 'relaxed' " (p. 6). In this state one may experience mental leaps between apparently unrelated thoughts. These "unexpected transitions" (p. 6) are the ground for metaphorical, analogic thinking that is fueled by affect linking. With this last term Gelernter indicates the impact of an affective state, that has reached an activated and experienced form, upon the process of thought formation and upon the link among various components of the entire thought process, as well as between these components and aspects of reality. Affect linking "brings together memories whose only connection is the particular emotion with which each is associated. Hence *"unexpected connections"* (p. 86). Gelernter also states that *"Not every affect link reveals a fact of scientific value, or of any practical value, but every affect link reveals a truth"* (p. 100; emphasis added).

Lowering of focus requires a diffuse state of attention rather than a sharply focalized state. While at high focus the thought process is very detailed and piercing, at low focus what comes forth is the entirety of a mental landscape. "The details and idiosyncrasies of the overlaid memories are simply blended. What emerges isn't a 'general principle,' but a new and idiosyncratic image" (p. 88). This new image may be what a creative insight consists of, and indeed Gelernter contends that a lowered focus state is crucial for the unfolding of the creative process.

In a significant passage of Gelernter's work I recognized the kernel to a central finding from my personal experience.

In substance, a high-focus thought-train tells you what
it is about . . . low-focus thought-streams . . . *don't* tell you
what they are about and this *not telling* is crucial to their
character . . . they are thematic, but their themes are
emotional themes . . . *there are no grounds for assuming
that the theme—the emotion that underpins the train and
gives it coherence—will appear at all in the version that has
been reduced to language.* (p. 32; emphasis added)

The importance of this conclusion in assessing the
outcomes of mental research is obvious: all reductionistic studies based on the exchange of purely verbal information or on a purely motoric response may completely
miss the theme that governs the entire mental process
under investigation.

Thought activity supported by high focus has been
essential for the development of the rational orientation and the scientific language and achievements that
have characterized the unfolding of the Western human
mind. However, there is a dark side to this mode of
thinking. As Gelernter puts it, "high-focus
thought . . . is literally unfeeling. Just because it is unfeeling, it excludes creativity and intuition and spirituality" (p. 65). He is of the opinion that spirituality resides
in a state of diffuse attention possible only at low focus:
"The essence of the phenomenon might be a sense of
connectedness" (p. 93).

Clearly, Gelernter speaks about a change in attention *and* about the role of affectivity upon recovery of
and linkage among memories (or, more broadly, stored
information). This view is consonant, to a point, with
my inner experience. What Gelernter's exploration
does not seem to address is the simultaneity and glob-
ality of the unconscious thinking that precedes the conscious, words formulated phase (see again his statement

quoted above). I claim that both low and high focus conscious thinking are constructed from a nonrepresentational and therefore nonconscious platform of global data elaboration (my very rapid thinking [VRT] mode). The linkages at this level happen out of felt, affectivity-based, gradients.

Hierarchical System

It envisions the nature of consciousness as closely related to a system of hierarchies of knowledge. Scott (1995) states:

> I propose . . . a metaphorical stairway . . . a hierarchy of mental organization in which most of us . . . unwittingly stand at the two top steps or levels, consciously aware of the realities of our culture. But the lower steps are every bit as important to our position at the uppermost level. . . . Thus, I suggest consciousness is an emergent phenomenon, one born of many discrete events fusing together as a single experience. (p. 3)

He then describes the hierarchical ladder as consisting, from the top down, of culture, consciousness, brain, assemblies of neurons, neurons, nerve impulses, biochemical structures, molecules and atoms. The dynamic laws that govern each level of the hierarchy are largely disconnected from each other. And these system dynamics are nonlinear in that the effect from the sum of the myriad of atomistic components of each layer is not equal to the sum of the individual effects. Scott states that "the whole is not equal to the sum of its parts. Nonlinearity is less convenient for the analyst because things can happen . . . —new atomistic building blocks may *emerge* at each hierarchical level—and that is why the realm of biology is so rich" (pp. 189–190).

The current book may also hold an epistemological value, as it incorporates several of the nine characteristics proposed in the paper by Harman (1996):

1. The epistemology will be "radically empirical" . . . (it will include subjective experience as primary data . . .) and it will address the totality of human experience. . . .

2. It will aim at being objective in the sense of being open and free from hidden bias, while dealing with both "external" and "internal" (subjective) experience as origins of data.

3. It will insist on open inquiry and public (intersubjective) validation of knowledge; at the same time it will recognize that these goals may, at any given time, be met only incompletely. . . .

4. It will place emphasis on the unity of experience. It will thus be congenial to a holistic view in which the parts are understood through the whole. . . .

5. It will recognize that science deals with models and metaphors representing certain aspects of experienced reality and that any model or metaphor may be permissible if it is useful. . . .

6. It will thus recognize the partial nature of all scientific concepts of causality . . . it will implicitly question the assumption that a nomothetic science—one characterized by inviolable "scientific laws"—can in the end adequately deal with causality.

7. It will be participatory in recognizing that understanding comes . . . from cooperating or identifying with the observed, and experiencing it subjectively. . . .

8. It will involve recognition of the inescapable role of the personal characteristics of the observer, including the processes and content of the unconscious mind . . . the researcher must be willing to risk being profoundly changed through the process of exploration.

9. Because of this . . . an epistemology that is accepted now may in time have to be replaced by another. . . . (pp. 747–748)

The data presented in the following pages are radically empirical; they couldn't be more so! They have been collected through an effort that was as much as possible open and free from hidden bias (there has been no drive to force them to fit a specific theoretical shape). A significant effort has been made to stimulate and facilitate intersubjective validation (the examples have been kept simple and common, to promote replicability). The experiences have been presented as gestalts, holistic and yet composed of parts. There is an ongoing effort to remind readers that all this is simply a model and that what I present is expressed through metaphors. And so on.

Maybe one day, I hope never, we may develop the ability to connect the human brain to a recording device that would register, analyze, interpret and understand all of a person's selfhood (sort of William James' super-automaton).[4] Such selfhood—the composite of the entire set of mental states constantly interacting, either through potential or actual links—could then be revealed and objectified.

It looks, though, as if the sheer immensity of the number of possible mental states will forever protect the ultimate privacy and individuality of the human mind.

Conclusions

Objective observations of mental function are limited to what the subject can communicate to an observer.

[4]James introduced and discussed an "automaton-theory," in which the brain was considered a complex machine operating through many reflexes of the spinal cord type and the mind became an epiphenomenon, only to conclude

These conscious observable mental acts are therefore expressed as motor events (a thought cannot be objectively observed unless it is expressed and shared through some sort of motor activity) that reflect the function of selected groups of neurons (networks), the equivalents of the "apple-web." These conscious acts follow the laws of classical physics.

Subjectivity, instead, represents the elaboration, for potential or actual use, of our entire set of knowledge. Subjective events are both conscious inner occurrences (thoughts, beliefs, emotions, values, and so on) and the nonconscious subliminal inner states that constitute our entire accumulation of information. The source of this "knowledge" will be postulated in the next chapter and presented in chapters 3 through 7. The knowledge is constantly interconnected and interactive in its entirety, it filters and assimilates the perceptions from the external world, and it arranges reality.

The interactive process is guided by affective states. This point will be presented in chapter 7. Affect linking may offer access to the entire set of mental landscapes. The sea of data that support our subjective experiencing forms the matrix from which mental choices eventually become visible in the realm of classical reality as conscious acts. This complex activity resides also in the brain, as neural networks do, but its site may be subneuronal, and its laws may belong to a nonclassical type of physics. The activity may consist of simultaneous, superimposed potential states, solutions, alternatives, possibilities and so on, which collapse at the synapse into specific neurochemical events. These events ultimately coalesce into the conscious act.

that "to urge the automaton-theory upon us . . . is an unwarrantable impertinence in the present state of psychology." (As cited in Scott [1995] pp. 106–107.) I suspect James would be of the same opinion even today.

So we have an objective, apparently replicable, conscious set of mental events and a subjective, conscious and nonconscious, set of mental organizations, permutable and ever changing. The use of the reductionistic replicable approach to specific neural sequences in studying the mind and consciousness will at best present us with shallow copies, as in the Guernica–Pietá metaphor. The subjective inner process needs to be accessed, accepted, and calculated in order to understand how brain and mind really work. The immense diversity of possible minds that could be obtained by different combinations of the neural and subneural dynamic structures is so great that individuality remains uncontested, and duplication of our selfhood impossible.

CHAPTER TWO

Two Mentalistic Portraits

> No intelligent man will dare to com-
> mit his philosophical thoughts to
> words, still less to *words that cannot be
> changed,* as is the case with what is
> expressed in written character.
> (Plato, 1973, p. 138; emphasis added)

The Book and Its Content

Plato's skepticism about the limitation of language in
teaching and disseminating knowledge sounds particularly appropriate when the theme consists of abstract,
subjective, and mentalistic material. Despite these reser-
vations, I will describe with words my thoughts and reflections concerning the structure of my mind and
(speculatively but likely) the structure of the human
mind in general.

I have previously indicated the scarcity of data on
subjectivity. The present book tries to address this
dearth of an information base. Its scientific objective is
a programmatic presentation of a robust set of carefully
assessed data on subjective mental content and mental
operations. The mental contents share the characteristic of having been experienced as gestalts, rather than
"reconstructed" through sequential associational work.
Increased understanding of the marked and critical difference between intuitive, simultaneous, mental activity

(characteristic of subjectivity), and conscious, sequential, analytical cognition (the ingredient of rational thought and objective studies), in my opinion would be a very significant contribution to a comprehensive science of the mind. Therefore the book gives special attention to the phenomenon of intuition and to the world of nonconscious mental states.

The data and the mental contents are traced back to known sources of *learning:* the genetic endowment of the species, its evolutionary developmental lines, and individualized experiential learning. The data are interpreted as representing the *emergent* product from these vast sources of mental knowledge.

The introspective method used in the following chapters to collect material illustrative of my subjective functioning does not suggest that introspection is the science of subjectivity. I merely used the only tool currently available for a systematic collection and description of the very complex dynamic structures that lie behind all processes of thought. For these structures I have chosen the term *gestalts* as the most descriptive label and I affirm that we need to deal with them (i.e., to develop a science of subjectivity) as a first step toward a true science of consciousness.

The book is based, therefore, on a process of self-disclosure. I will use a series of personal examples to illustrate the pervasive quality of unconscious processes and unconscious awareness, my genetic endowment, my system of values, the fabric of my qualia,[1] and the role of intentionality, my quantum relationship to other realities. In the process I will also suggest how all these

---

[1] I use the term *qualia* to indicate the basic unit of experience just as quanta are the basic units of matter. See also the following section on the world of affects, emotions, and the qualia.

elements may influence my concept formation, concept elaboration, and memory. And I will discuss my subjective perception of a multilayered system of thought development and the role played by the use of symbols and of language.

The selection criteria for these personal examples was kept simple, to represent true common grounds and to evoke similar themes from the reader's gestalts. The data are presented *as they happen to emerge* without conscious attempt to manipulate them into fitting a specific hypothesis (this neutrality represents a true challenge for the researcher of the subjective). The assessment of the different gestalts is fundamentally *intuitive* (as the gestalts are themselves), i.e., based on what I call the process of *very rapid thinking* (VRT). With this term I refer to the vast and simultaneous activation of the entire set of data that are, in any and all possible ways, related to the mental task. Given the global affective (qualia-based?) interconnectivity of my "library of knowledge" (aside from the possible quantal mode of function of this phase in thought formation), it is likely that the entire library becomes activated in toto. Such simultaneous availability and elaboration of experiential, inherited, and affective data allows for the synchronous coexistence of multiple solutions. Of these, a finite number will eventually collapse into concrete representational constructs that intuitively emerge into consciousness as *relational thinking* (RT).[2] The VRT

---

[2]With this term I refer to the elaboration into consciousness of selected emergent products from the entire VRT process involved in a specific mental task. While, in my opinion, VRT is largely nonrepresentational, RT on the contrary is generally expressed in symbols, in structured and recognizable concepts that allow for both internal and external conscious communication and action. However, I suspect that RT may also occur in nonrepresentational, or at least nonconscious, states. The encounter with the antelope described in chapter 4 is an example of such states. In this case there was relatedness and complex relational behaviors were activated, but there was no conscious aware-

data are therefore different from the emergent, conscious end product, and in this sense the VRT concept
resembles the fringe concept of William James, and may
include the "vague" realm that he considered a major
component of mind. It is, however, my contention that
these states are (at least in part) susceptible to being
not only experienced but also described. In my opinion
the VRT process constitutes the foundation for all mental functioning.

I will then pair these personal experiences with vignettes largely taken from my clinical practice. Through
these I will borrow from the minds of others more extreme examples of my points (or, at least, what appear
to be examples of these points; the ultimate subjective
meaning at the basis of the vignettes naturally escaped
me, as my ultimate subjectivity would escape all the
readers of this book).

The concept of trying to respect the "mental functioning as it comes" is very important throughout the
book. I have tried to bring the readers into my psychological activity "through the kitchen," almost unexpectedly, and observe casual aspects of the "house"—the
unfinished cup of coffee, the fresh herbs on the
counter, peripheral subdivisions in my stream of
thoughts, shifting images of my subjective self.[3] For this
reason the vignettes are described as an active experience unfolding around me, rather than a mere recollection from the past. To me this approach to the
subjective is more fitting than the preorganized, sequential approach to consciousness in which the themes are

---

ness of what was being exchanged or of the language used to exchange such
"what."

    [3]These culinary images are not simple metaphors! As the text will show they
may truly represent specific aspects of my subjective landscapes.

presented from the external observer's point of view. The latter is a method that characterizes most of the current organized thought on mental functioning. I have tried instead to create a different study design that would allow for a different perception of the qualia, values, and organization of the mental household in its spontaneous existence and in its continuous balancing and readjusting acts.

The reader should be able to find each time something unique and yet familiar which is shared among the various parts of the book. He or she will learn to identify the infrastructure, the foundation themes that may define and organize the entirety of my subjective mental landscapes (and which inexorably determine its unreplicable uniqueness). The reader may skip a theme, or go to it later, or revisit at any time. To facilitate the reading of this material I will outline below the processes and data that will be considered throughout the book as well as my understanding of them. In the second section of this chapter I will specify the source of the data by offering an abbreviated outline of my development and of the major factors that contributed to molding such development.

Selfhood and Subjectivity

Selfhood and subjectivity represent the anchoring themes of the book. They comprise the exquisitely personal sense of selfhood; the variegated and dynamic landscape that constitutes who I am; its life-pulsating vastness beyond the shifting beam of consciousness; the certitude of my uniqueness and the constant, profound subjective coloring of all that happens and is. Beyond words, this coloring contains an experience of extreme individuation (even from an imaginary identical twin). Despite the spatial and temporal vastness of living creation, my wholeness simply cannot be found in others. It cannot be duplicated.

I operate and think in the isolation of my uniqueness, of my exclusive subjective space-time; other minds and selves are their own subjective mysteries within shells, my mental evocation of their true essence (but not of their meanings to me!) standing incomplete and minute, when compared to the gestalt of my selfhood.

And yet, when a living object enters my awareness, a sudden communion bursts into existence, by which I think, I know, I perceive, I capture some of the object's essence (empathy, spiritual communion, appreciation, "being touched," illusion, and so on). What a delightful paradox: a quintessential subjectivity that appears to have the potential for universal linkage!

Consciousness and the Unconscious

Consciousness is used as conscious awareness, in an elastic approximation of two states that probably have different neural organizations. Consciousness is like a great light cast upon the landscape of my essence: bright and sharply defined at the center of the beam; progressively dimmer and crepuscular and blurred and shifting in its images as it enters the penumbra at the periphery of the field. In that realm the transition to my unconscious ceaselessly repeats itself; and these two aspects continuously change in content and in their reciprocal balance. The unconscious always vastly prevails along the dimensions of my individual space-time, rich in life and experience. I sense its ongoing presence and vastness, as I would be aware of an unseen continent beyond the confines of my horizon. Indeed, often consciousness appears simply to be the elaboration into interactive symbolization of cognitive processes that happen in the unconscious state. Consciousness translates unconscious very rapid thinking (VRT) into relational thinking (RT); worded thoughts, words, movements, emotional expressions. Their use is to communicate both internally as well as externally. Examples of this process are presented in chapter 3. The process itself is summarized in Figure 1.2 (p. 16).

The Genetic Endowment

This genetic intelligence represents the substrate to and the product of evolutionary continuity and adaptation. I refer here not as much to the genetic machinery that promotes and guides organ development, protein synthesis, mutational potential, time and stress driven cascades of gene activation, and the like. Rather, I refer to the complex, intentional programs of adaptive interaction with the world that represent the true ultimate objective of evolutionary development. These are programs we recognize and share with nonhuman minds. They appear to be characterized by well-tested and preprogrammed behavioral responses (instincts?) that incorporate the capability for individual variations through multiple differences in the core general design. So the impala stag striving to establish its own form of selfhood would follow the shared genetic program of literally "locking horns" with the opponent. Don't we empathically, intuitively recognize the visceral significance of such behavior? But then individualized options would immediately emerge, dictated by the seriousness

of the challenge, the diversity in dominance and reciprocal respect, the importance of territorial statements.
The stag may continue the fight, or chose evasive action,
or pursue to a greater or lesser extent the evading opponent. All these individualized decisions may in turn trigger neurohormonal realignments and further
behavioral as well as true phenotypic changes (in the
impala, a shift in the dominance hierarchy may stimulate changes in the symmetry and shape of the stag's
horns). In humans these programs continue to play
leading roles. They have been subjected to species-specific modifications, but they also have retained a common paleogenetic substrate, susceptible to activation by
uncommon circumstances.

Furthermore, the genetic endowment contains indi-
vidual-oriented programs as well as species-oriented (social) ones, the two sets (or networks, or neuronal
"assemblies") being at times in opposition and differen-
tially weighted.[4]

I have come to the opinion that inherited knowledge
is organized in three layers, or orders. These layers probably differ not only in the content of the data, but also
in the form, the "language" in which the data have
been encoded and stored and, therefore, the manner
in which they are expressed. Layer 1 pertains to all the
major adaptive (mental) modes of interaction with the
environment that evolved prior to the differentiation of

---

[4]I use this term in the sense discussed by Hebb (1949), who suggested that
groups of neurons communicating with each other do not do so in a random
way. Rather, the operation of communication is facilitated by the process of
learning. Synaptic systems that interact with each other will continue to communicate in a preferential way, by developing stronger and easier links among
themselves. Such strengthening of communication among interrelated neurons
is also reminiscent of Edelman's concept of *synaptic metastability* that indicates
neuronal groups reversibly stabilized by synaptic connections primed through
the sharing of common functions and of specific biochemical processes.

the hominids. Its source of information may span from 300 million years ago (with the appearance of the mammal-reptiles of which we still carry brain components) to 10 to 5 million years ago and the origin of the hominids. Layer 2 relates to learned and discovered themes of dynamic adaptation to the environment from the dawn of the species, from the *australopithecinae* to *Homo habilis* and *Homo erectus* and eventually *sapiens*. Its source of information spans from 5 million years ago to less than 10,000 years ago and the origin of the first protocultures. Layer 3 is concerned with the narrower component of derivative mental programs of adaptation that came to be elaborated by the sociocultural themes present in the ancestral line. This layer may cover learning from the last few millennia. The presence of this material in my subjective system is exemplified in chapters 4 through 6.

Systems of Values and Needs, Intrinsic and Acquired

Intrinsic and acquired systems of values and needs are the ongoing determinants and modifiers of the orientation and content of my consciousness and of my unconscious mental activity. To all of us it comes as an intuitive given that such systems be universally shared as common, species-adapted themes, but that they also assume in each one of us an exquisitely unique, individualized organization, and a balance of subtle priorities and preferences, that reflect both the inheritance of the collective experience from our ancestors and our exclusive individual experience with life. As an example, we all share an instinctive understanding of territoriality (that is probably why we understand the behavior of the impala). We also have reached our particular, idiosyncratic representation of the territorial issue, through its inter-action and realignment with the entirety of our individ-ualized system of values.

In other words, the data contained in the accumu-lated set of genetic "books" modified through eons, that eventually became the template of our species, un-dergo progressive elaboration through the evolution of our individual lineage. Along these "ancestors lines" the original messages have acquired further differentia-tion through the collective experiential learning of the lineage. Experiential learning has increased exponen-tially, as the history of tool development illustrates in a dramatic way. The flour (prehuman level) and the yeast (protohuman level) are the same: the leavening and the molds reflected different values and expectations.

All these data are then processed through our indi-vidual experiential learning: the frostings, the changes in oven temperature, the choices in seasonings. There-fore, while one could apply stochastic rules to these en-sembles and deduct stochastic similarities among their phenomenological outcomes, the unreplicable and ob-jectively out-of-reach individuality of our selfhood is glaringly beyond discussion. Imagine the complexity of all these data being processed along the global vastness of an individual human brain as reflected in the im-mense numbers of possible mental states mentioned earlier in the text. How could such a set be duplicated? Examples of this material and its impact on mental func-tions are given in chapters 5 and 6.

The Worlds of Affects, Emotions, and the Qualia

In the vast realm of feeling states words have indeed an overall limited clarifying role. I will generally, but not religiously, use the term *affect* to indicate a communicable elaboration of an emotional state: the component that colors the cognitive counterpart and that is somewhat identifiable and recognizable by an observer. The word *emotion* (feeling) indicates my inner experience, the *motus animi;* not always developed to the point of allowing for a label nor for external, and internal, recognition; but clearly, although indescribably, a composite and elaborate product of experiences and exposures. *Qualia* is a term that helps me to share my suspicion that emotions are indeed the complicated end-products of more elemental bits of affective experience that are imbedded in the (subjective) attributes of all the mental objects participating in my internal reality. Emotions are the summation and the emergent result of temporally distinct and qualitatively different qualia of experience.[5] Metaphorically the qualia are the notes, the emotion is the tune, the affect is the audience-oriented performance of the symphony, vested with a cognitive meaning and a title. The roles of affectivity and of intentionality (the next topic in this list) are described and exemplified in chapter 7.

Intentionality

Behind all aspects of creation and being lurks a subtle underlying raison d'être, possibly all the way down to the elusive potentialities of quantum phenomena. This concept of intentional states is greatly elaborated by Searle (1993). The presence of a content and of its conditions of satisfaction (and, sporadically, the related

---

[5]In a personal communication, Nick Herbert comments how "one of the biggest steps forward in mind science would be the discovery and measurement of the units and numerical value of this purported quantum of subjectivity."

generation of a happening) characterizes all mental states and mental machinery. We operate along a vast fabric of intertwined intentional states that originate shimmering images of potential resolutions, and occasionally eventuate in specific affairs. Searle (1992) also affirms that all intentional states always have an aspectual shape. He uses this term, borrowed from the visual arts, to indicate that "whenever we perceive anything or think about anything, we always do so under some aspects and not others" (pp. 156–157). Searle also contends that "these aspectual features are essential to the intentional state: *They are part of what makes it the mental state that is*' " (p. 157; emphasis added). He illustrates how during our interaction with various configurations of reality "something is believed or desired about them only under certain aspects and not under others. Every belief and every desire, and indeed every intentional phenomenon, has an aspectual shape" (p. 157). Such aspectual shape, such pervasive frame of reference, is inherently subjective, as the examples from my clinical cases confirm. Furthermore, the concept implies that all our mental operations, or events, are always affected at their origin by this frame of reference.

The foundation of Searle's hypothesis of Intentionality consists of the concepts of *Background* and *Network*. Intentional networks require an elaborate background set of "capacities, abilities and general know-how that enable our mental states to function" (p. 196). The Background therefore refers to the entire spectrum of brain structures and activities, from the subcellular to the neural. An illustration of Background activity may be my apple-web.

Quantum Mechanics and Mental Function

Maybe we simply need an occasional escape from classical reality in order to dream and to speculate on a more intimate connectedness with the marvels of the universe, from the very large to the very small. Still, the whimsical qualities of quantum physics—where magic becomes a mathematical truth, and space-time a sandbox for creations and dissolutions—may indeed justify, eventually, some of humanity's inborn curiosity and belief in universality and in the expansiveness of the human mind outside of the boundaries of classical reality. And although the potentiality of quantum structures appears to be by definition not observable, still I will attempt to share vibrations from other dimensions that appear occasionally to tinge my classical inner world: weird and yet numinous variations in the perception of all that is, as well as in the formation of concepts. These shadows of uncertain realities and entangled possibilities (or probabilities) may indeed represent the subjective accurate experience of quantum physical events that may precede the classical neurophysiological phenomena underlying my selfhood and consciousness. The correlation between the physics of the quantum world and the processes of the mind is examined in chapter 8.

The Author: A Vastly Condensed Version

I will now introduce an outline of some core developmental themes and motifs from experiential learning that probably played an influential role in orienting and shaping into my specific singularity the collective, archetypal material that had been progressively elaborated during the evolution of the species and of my ancestry. In this way my unique mind came into being by means of the interplay between knowledge of old and my experiencing of life.[6]

I am an only child. My two ancestral lines and families were interestingly organized along complementary patterns. The two families had superficially similar but structurally diverse interests and, to some extent, value systems that overall were compatible and reciprocally supportive.

My paternal family was truly paternal; it was largely male in its themes and in its predominant configurations. Men formed its glue and motif; landowners, merchants, and lawyers, they maintained a rather conservative hold on estates and business, the family library, the decor of the homes, the relationship with the local community. My global memory is that of a sturdy, dependable, massive-walled, emotionally constricted although not cold gestalt. There were large empty dark spaces, dust, and the practice of avoiding unnecessary sounds, both in a concrete and in a metaphorical sense. My maternal family was, in contrast, characterized by glittering male figures who were clearly expressions of their women. Themes, properties, choices, careers, homes, they were all decided and designed by the women, and their men's achievements, while graciously acknowledged and praised, were unquestionably known to belong in reality to the women, the true muses of the system. My global impression is

---

[6]A rich exploration of the archetypal world can be found in all Jungian depth psychology. Equally profound studies concerning the organization of the individualized psychic structures characterizes Freudian and post-Freudian psychology. It is telling of human functioning that these complementary psychological schools have often been at odds with each other.

that of a tastefully sensuous, intense, artistic, permutable but always stylish gestalt.

I was born in Eritrea, then an Italian colony in East Africa, along the Red Sea, and became one of the first casualties of World War II when "for safety reasons" it was decided that my mother and I should return to Italy to wait for the end of what was anticipated to be a short war. I was 2 years old and did not see my father again for over 6 years.

Those were years of profound changes and severe deprivation, marked by the collapse of what had for generations been a stable way of gentry living. They were years of suffering and grieving, constant sounds of war and daily devastation, in a world devoid of men and run by women fiercely struggling to maintain values and for the literal survival of themselves and their children.

My second decade of life literally started with our return to Africa. This event had the most profound impact on the development of my mind by offering me the richness of vast contrasts, in practical terms extremes of very complex ranges of experience, at an age when nothing had as yet been crystallized, but the magic and the molding and the adaptation were still easy and natural. I grew up during those years in Eritrea at 9,000 feet above sea level, on the peak of a mountain enveloped by space and immense, open skies, in a small Italianlike town surrounded by untouched landscapes, as alien from the Italian ones as the customs of its people were from the ones I had left behind.

Very early, I remember, I began to realize these differences and to reflect on them. Theories about humanity and values were daily challenged by these different realities and showed their inadequacies and tentativeness. These challenges to my tradition were complex to integrate and could have been disturbing and confusing, had it not been that I was carrying within me the experience of an incredibly savage and destructive war, and of challenges and changes vastly superior, and more malevolent than the ones I was now presented with. These last ones were exciting, and liberating.

Furthermore the world that surrounded me was permeated with magic and unspoiled beauty, and with a nurturing, common (primeval?) spirituality linking all aspects of nature. Such a world spoke directly to the senses and to a part of me that responded to strange calls and felt familiarity (a very peculiar sense of déjà vu) with this untouched Nature, the animism that permeated it, the magic and the language of its nonhuman creatures, and its essential simplicity and symmetry.

It became simple to me as a young adolescent to move, without apparent effort and transition, from the moist, warm, spicy, naked and very sensuous experiences of the native bazaars to the ritualized, controlled, intelligent and stimulating, prudish home environment. I distinctly remember being aware that these two worlds were separate and that I should not challenge them to assimilate for my benefit; and yet being fully able to live in and enriched by both sets of experience.

A third and very important event for my psychological development followed my father's decision to leave the city and go to manage a vast cotton plantation at the Eritrea–Sudan border. I was by then in my late teens. The place he moved to was the real Africa, at the end of distant roads that turned from tar to gravel and then to sand. While traveling along such roads not only did the imported Italian remnants of our Western system progressively disappear, but also the very traces of humanity became tenuous and ephemeral. I spent long periods of great spiritual beauty in those millions of acres of uninhabited savanna and in the dense palm forests along the huge, mostly dry, river that at the end of each rainy season in the highlands would flood the cotton fields. I would become truly immersed in the marvels of nature. The complete absence of any trace of humanity allowed me, as never before or after, to feel in a sense less human and more "life-being." I touched wildlife and was touched by it, without effort; and I had a clear glimpse at the feeling that made men find spirits in trees and rocks and in the planet itself. It was the same experience of original religion ("pietas") in the sense that Lucretius (1992) gives to the word.[7] Such profound communion with creation, and the sharp awareness of a common language, has never left me and still represents the nucleus to which I turn when I search for inner harmony. These were indeed the roots of the simplicity in approaching change, the curiosity and the comfort about newness and complementary opposites that have stimulated and facilitated the multiple pere-grinations that have characterized a large part of my professional and adult life.

I eventually moved to Milan to finish medical school. The difference was very profound. Every day each expe-rience was a source of curiosity and reflection. Having failed for financial and pragmatic reasons to start my psychiatric training in Italy, I moved to Nigeria (a very magical country, where men could turn into goats after sunset while carrying Bibles in their pockets and lust in

---

[7]Nec pietas illast vellatum saepe videri—vertier ad lapidem atque omnis accedere ad aras . . . sed mage placata posse omnia mente tueri." (It is not piety to show oneself often with covered head—turning toward a stone and approaching every altar . . . but rather to be able to look with a tranquil mind at the immensity of creation) (pp. 470–471).

their intentions); and I stayed there for 5 years. I practiced literally every aspect of medicine; I directed my own missionary hospital, and developed a private practice. I got married and we had two children.

My North American experience began with what I had anticipated to be a 2- to 3-year period of training before returning to missionary medicine. During the next 2 years I became very immersed in brain structure, and aware of the abyss between the scalpel and the mind. As my English improved I began to attend psychiatric events in New Haven, and realized that indeed I could try to attain what had eluded me in Italy.

I started training in psychiatry, and this became the most significant anchoring factor to my new country. The choice was symbolically expressed by my relinquishing my Italian citizenship and becoming an American citizen during my second year of psychiatric residency. The shift had been facilitated by my having driven across the country and having realized that I still had a wonderful, profoundly diverse, and fascinating continent to explore, in a culture that considered internal migrations as an ordinary human condition.

Over the next two decades I was fortunate in finding professional opportunities that allowed me to programmatically continue to concentrate on the systematic observation of human subjective experiences. My professional activity kept me exposed to human minds as these minds gradually communicated some of their hidden landscapes. Many of these exposures were allowed to proceed at a great depth, a depth usually left unexplored, or actually unknown, by the usual patterns of mental interaction (indeed, the experience of a naked mind is so unusual that most people find it acutely embarrassing, and rush to cloak it with proper superficiality). The diversity of subjects that has characterized my clinical practice furnished a wide spectrum of idiosyncratic mental states. In these clinical cases collective themes often appeared to have suffered from distortions caused by the impact of epigenetic or early developmental pathological experiences.[8] Frequently these minds appeared to operate along a spectrum of complex subjective realities more or less set apart from the reality of the observer. My academic role included the need to discuss with others these minds and their ways of operating. This need enhanced my skill in formulating reasonable metaphors that would resonate empathically in my students and carry some true images of all these subjective landscapes.

In my free time I have of late cherished a unique relationship that is truly magical and eternal in its origin. In my other free time, among other things I tend flowers and plants; and somewhat leisurely, I reflect on the relationship that the mind has with life and the universe. I have great fun at that.

Conclusions

The method followed in this search is atheoretical. I used spontaneous, immediate self-disclosure of the data and processes (related to a conscious mental act) that I appeared to capture intuitively within my mind.

My self-concept is quite unique and unreplicable, but has also significant empathic "familiarity" to others.

---

[8] In some cases of inherited or at least familial "psychopathology" the development of the individual self could be jeopardized by dysfunctional programs directing the unfolding of "brute" neural structures as well as by the inheritance of maladaptive or inappropriate collective themes.

This connectedness seems to emerge from some unknown inner space or process and to exist at the periphery of consciousness: it is a nonrepresentational state,
until described to the self and to the observer.

While individual experiential learning differentiates
us from each other, what I call genetic intelligence creates intuitive bridges of recognition and commonality
among us.

By genetic intelligence I refer primarily to inherited
programs of behavioral adaptation to the external
world[9] rather than to the better known genetic programs geared to the development of the physical structure. Thus we recognize postures and behaviors that
came into being in order to define territorial needs, or
dominance messages. We inherit adaptive styles that
had emerged even before the evolution of our species,
at the dawn of life.

These ancient adaptive programs developed into inner states that we now label as needs or values, and that
affect each single act of perception. These states had a
very ancient common origin; they then branched out in
several elaborations dictated by different evolutionary
collective directions (or cultures) and became finally
further modified by individual experience.

Therefore inherited knowledge is conceptualized in
layers: Layer 1 data were collected before the differentiation of the *hominoideae;* layer 2 data were common to
hominoid's evolution; layer 3 data were related to more
recent racial and sociocultural characteristics.

---

[9]The behavioral ecologist Marc Hauser from Harvard points to the significant role of adaptationist thinking in many areas of psychological research.
Psychologist Steve Pinker from MIT suggests that "our emotions were shaped
by our evolutionary environment, not the one we grew up in" (see N. Williams,
1997a). And evolutionary biologist Helena Cronin at the London School for
Economics studies the effect of cultural factors and evolution in the shaping
of mental functions (see N. Williams, 1997b).

The driving impetus of these states is given by the affective weight and by their intentional coefficient. Affectivity and intentionality are the common attributes of these states, and a key to pull them into consciousness. They possibly operate as quantum states.

The history of my personal selfhood reflects these themes:

1. Long "ancestor lines" where stereotyped searches for "the right way" eventuated in the formation of complementary systems that could coexist, despite their intrinsic diversity, because they shared the common template of the larger cultural group.

2. The theme of opposites ran in a consistent fashion throughout my early individual learning: the opposites of a war, of two countries and their two cultures, habits, and value systems. Possibly all this inherited and acquired experience stirred a search for and curiosity about diversity and opposites, and mastery in negotiating coexistence and identifying common themes.

3. The African experience came at a very crucial developmental period and acted as a counterpoint to the previous war experience, acquiring therefore a very positive affective value. Its prevailing magical and natural characteristics probably enhanced my capacity for affect linking and for heightened resonance with nature and paleohuman or nonhuman life.

4. Themes and experiences of vast spaces relatively immune from the dimension of time found a reflection in the largely spatial orientation of my psychic inner world.

My prolonged professional exposure to mental phenomena and function attests that I have achieved a substantial sophistication in searching for subjective landscapes and evaluating them. The same professional exposure counts for my above average level of programmatic learning about the intuitive process and the familiarity phenomenon. In other words, I can be considered a scientist in these areas.

CHAPTER THREE

Workings of the Mind: Consciousness and the Unconscious

> I have always found in my own work
> . . . that zeroing tightly on a particular
> problem is self-defeating. Why not re-
> lax . . . and our unconscious mind . . .
> may solve the problem for [us].
> (Janov Pelorat, as quoted by Asimov,
> 1991b, p. 109)

A Personal Vignette: "Finding the Road"

On an overcast August Saturday afternoon, while scattered showers appear from nowhere deterring
beachgoers with their inconsistency, route 28 in Fal-
mouth, Massachusetts, is an unknown and frustrating
road to drive along. There is nowhere to park, and driving is a constant refocusing of attention and tapping at
the steering column. Marion would like to find where
she had lived, for a momentous year, three decades ago.
She recalls a lake, a street—Lakeside drive, or could it
be Lakeview drive? Our two maps are of no help, adding
only further clutter to the interior of our car.

As I drive I take critical notice of the ubiquitous,
unappealing taste of the stereotypical tourists. I also
keep a skeptical eye open for the improbable mirage of
a parking space, and build fantastic hidden meanings

out of the many car plates surrounding us: playful analogies that capture their unaware owners in a lattice of
connectedness and profound, although brief and
ephemeral, reciprocal significance. Marion's search is
by now very peripheral to my mental landscape, almost
in the penumbra of the nonconscious; only polite love
keeps it silhouetted in the distance.

And then I hear myself say, "Ask a real estate agent."

I instantly realize that I have never thought that!
Naturally, it is a very appropriate option and will indeed
be the successful move. (We found the street, and the
lake, and the house, and old neighbors of 30 years before.) But I *did not think* it. I do not think about real
estate persons or agencies. I am rather unfamiliar with
them; Marion is more at ease in dealing with that
world—but it was not she who thought the solution!

What happened to these two minds differently activated by the same task? I cannot and do not want to
speak for the other mind; I will simply speculate on
some reasonable differences between the two, and then
go on with my own mental processes.

For a start, I had never been in that area before,
either in a concrete or in an abstract, metaphorical way.
Thirty years ago, I did not know Marion. I had not yet
come to this country, I did not have any memory of the
landscape that she was trying to reconstruct: I had not
driven those roads, looked at the lake surrounded by
the magic of its woods at sunset, in the New England
fall. She had tried to describe it to me but evidently her
words could not paint her subjective images in my mind.
I had not been exposed to the life-shattering event that
had befallen her; I had not felt the shimmer of the
morning light on that lake merging with the shimmer
of love from another presence. I had been told of a

house and a porch on the water and a path to it, and I had once looked at a snapshot of yellow walls and unknown faces, but with gentle inattention, without really seeing it.

I can also speculate that she was probably at a level of focused attention different from mine. In a loose way, our mental configurations reflected what Gelernter (1994) describes as high and low focus states: "high focus thought (is) numb . . . literally unfeeling . . . excludes creativity and intuition and spirituality . . . is . . . adaptive . . . its huge power is obvious" (pp. 65–66). "As focus falls, attention becomes more diffuse. No single point . . . is sharply illuminated. It is consistently singled out as *the* mental state that gives rise to creativity or inspiration" (pp. 15–16). Marion wouldn't need to search for the house; she would have no problem in recognizing it, her first home, once she got there. She was therefore highly focused on the search for "a place": a lake, a street. Such places are found on maps, and her attention was narrowed to the map: probing, analyzing each street against old memories of names and traveled routes. She was probably too focused, too conscious, and her narrow beam of attention locked out the unconscious work of the mind.

I was, on the contrary, in a sort of idle problem-solving mode. My attention was underfocused, scattered among several mental processes. The futility of trying to solve the traffic or the parking and the impinging of all those people upon my unwilling sensory system shifted me to a low level of engagement with the environment. Subliminally fed up, I began to play with environmental cues, possibly as a way of diffusing my frustrated state and as a mild retaliation. The game then evoked people in their places; possibly places where people live; a desire to get out of the present reality; the peripheral but persisting, low-keyed awareness of Marion's ongoing task, that kept us involved; the tenuously conscious wish that she (we) would find the house (the only image pertaining to the task that would be present in my mind, from those old photographs, and even that one rather vague and indistinct); and—now fully nonconscious—memories of other times when Marion and I went searching for a house to make into our first home, the same emotion of wanting the search to succeed, being moderately fed up by then with realtors and they with us.

Was this what happened? I reexamined, almost immediately, the entire sequence: I had been really puzzled and surprised by the brilliant certainty of my complete lack of any conscious ownership of that mental product and I kept returning to explore it and probe it for its hidden meanings and origins. To me it represented a striking example of a routine, nonconscious, "intuitive" process. I could easily recollect some of its ingredients: my low level of conscious attention, my frustration, and yet my desire to help in the task, the prevailing, nameless moods that accompanied the flow of playful analogies. But the other crucial memories of similar and yet dissimilar scenes were, at those first reviews, totally hidden and remained so until I deliberately lowered my attention level and just allowed my thoughts to be suspended in a vague field in which the sequence itself would pulsate only in an intermittent fashion. Then those specific, linking, analogy-oriented memories suddenly "turned up" and they instantaneously "made sense." All this material had been processed in its totality, out of consciousness, and then a composite outcome, a thought, suddenly appeared from nowhere into my consciousness.

Is this the real story? Although the topic is my mind with its thought processes, I know that I cannot answer this question in any proven way. I can only decide or not to accept the explanation (which is also "unconscious-generated") trusting that somewhere in me I may indeed have the ability to reach some understanding of what my thoughts are about. The hidden mental system that originated a correct answer to the Cape Cod search may again be relied upon to produce the right explanation for its own functioning. Indeed, and this is the theme of this book, I am coming to the conclusion that my subjective understanding of my mental processes is by far superior to any and all speculative reconstruction by scientific "observers."

The vastness of the concealed, secret territory surrounding, directing, and propelling mental outcomes and products into the narrow field of my conscious awareness has at times a truely numinous quality. No wonder that so many thinkers have described the roots of the self and of the human mind through so many complex and deep-layered metaphors. I too have become filled with great awe when facing the ever-changing interaction between the conscious and the unconscious states of my mental landscape. As with so many others, I have felt deeply the fascination of the process of consciousness and of its generative background and counterpoint, unconsciousness. My clinical work has intensively nourished such wonderment and curiosity, through innumerable exposures to altered states of consciousness and to the profound variability among states, from state to state, and within each state. The opening clinical vignette in the Introduction, as well as the ones that will follow, amply illustrate such variability.

Edelman (1989) describes consciousness as "the remembered present." Susan Greenfield (1995) and others have tried different global definitions. I still struggle with the boundaries, the link between consciousness and selfhood; with the dynamics and their secret science of the interplay between these two states, and the role, the positioning of the concept of selfhood within the entire gestalt of the mind.

I struggle because, in my case, whenever "I am" I need to be in some form of conscious state, the dream state being possibly at one extreme of the spectrum of selfhood awareness. Yet I am quite aware that I am more than consciousness; but at any one time I can only observe so much; at any one time the field of my consciousness can contain only a limited set of my mental gestalt. Scouting my psychic universe can illuminate and decode scene upon scene, but for each one that enters my awareness another one fades away[1] out of conscious attention, its energy and value still as operative as before, its connections with the surrounding realm still preserved, but maybe now in a very different psychophysical state, free from representational obligations.

As noted in an earlier chapter, for my own benefit and clarity I refer to these nonrepresentational states as very rapid thinking (VRT) states.[2] They portray for me

---

[1] In a paper by David Galin (1994) on awareness, I recently found a very similar statement by psychologist B. Mangan (1991): "For something to become clear, something else must become vague" (p. 117). Here, as in many other places, I simply reinstate personal experiences that seem to have received a high degree of "intersubjective validation."

[2] These states will be discussed again in chapter 7. My VRT concept parallels to a point the fringe concept of James, but not fully. For instance, VRT does not include only "feelings of rightness" and the like, but also complex multilayered gestalts.

the *immense* number of mental configurations that constellate my individual space-time and that are instantaneously available even in response to very limited cues, very narrow demands, or very trivial stimuli. I may at times perceive a flash of these states, particularly when I spread my field of consciousness by diminishing conscious attention or during states of enhanced affectivity. At these moments, I grasp glimpses of such nonlocal and nonrepresentational activity pulsating all around, like flames or whirls of fog at the consciousness-horizon of my mental landscape. Such a landscape is life itself; my process of being alive; my process of being.

By contrast, consciousness[3] appears to be a state based upon the need to communicate, both internally and with the external environment. Consciousness and some aspects of self-identity are communicative devices: the global translation of the collapsed outcomes from VRT activity into relational thinking (RT): transferable, understandable packets of information, environmentally recognizable.

The data emerging from nonconscious work are coded into operational, rational structures. "Now I understand": I can now proceed, and further elaborate these data into semantic products that respond to rules and are applicable in classical reality, and ultimately communicable to others. I can use them to solve the problem—after all that is why they were furnished to "me" in the first place. I can narrow my attention to a pinpoint, and focus exclusively on selected data and

---

[3]I do not refer here to the basic, structural level of consciousness that distinguishes the presence of mental operations and that disappears under anesthesia or when the brain stops functioning but is not dead yet. Rather, I refer to functional conscious and unconscious processes and states, both within the operational model of being mentally alive.

sequentially elaborate their message and utility, while adding further analogic information that continues to emerge from the VRT level and to support my problem-solving condition.

I am indeed aware that the less attentive I am, the larger my perceived mental landscape becomes. However, the focus becomes less precise, the images dim and ambivalent, shimmers of potential holograms rather than sharp realistic configurations. They may be quite vivid as in dreams, but their logic is polymorphic and evanescent. Their themes are life itself and the emotional drives that constitute life's energy.

I need to clarify that I do not consider attention as the separator between consciousness and unconsciousness, between a focus and a penumbra of VRT activity. Attention plays a role in affect linking, and attention dimming may be essential to bring VRT activity into consciousness. But dimming is not essential to VRT activity per se. I am talking about consciousness, not attention. I will return to these experiences and their relationship with emotions in chapter 7.

So I still struggle. On one side I am sharply aware that my self representation requires my consciousness of it (what Edelman calls higher order consciousness, or the process of being "conscious of being conscious"). On the other hand I am equally sharply aware that most of my selfhood is mostly unconscious, most of the time.

In a certain way these concepts—consciousness, unconsciousness, selfhood—are but different names for the same mental structures. When these structures respond to different intentionalities they appear to organize themselves differently. So, selfhood I perceive as my entire space-time of experiences; my conscious self-image (my imago? my persona?) is the expression of an interactive state, either internally or externally, that requires a skeletal nucleus from the selfhood global identity to support a situational, much more limited and "local" appearance and presentation.[4]

Amusingly I reflect how my inner self representation is not truly ageless, but conveniently set on an undetermined but lesser age point than the one that characterizes my classical reality. A somehow optimal compromise for which I get older more slowly than in real time and yet I am not too young either. The subjective time sequence is different from the objective sequence. Such inner, exquisitely subjective balance is truly the most functional and adaptive for me, as it has kept me in a "best" place of being, experiencing and acting through the multiple changes that have punctuated my living experience.

An Objective Example: "The Silicon Pretender"

In mid-February 1996 some of us stood anxiously watching a champion of human creativity, Gary Kasparov, wrestle for the exclusiveness of the human mind with a purely algorithmic creature, Deep Blue, that could unfold a neural web covering hundreds of miles from Philadelphia to its crucial computational thinking center in Yorktown Heights, New York. At both ends of this web a score of humans—technicians, coaches, electronic masseuses—appeared to be continuously involved in

---

[4]We all have different self-images, with their distinct identities. As examples, the parental, the professional, the lover self-images are different from each other in substantial ways. We enter them in response to environmental situations.

loving ministrations (somewhat reminiscent, to me, of bees around a queen), to keep the flow of algorithmic knowledge that would assess, back and forth, an average of 100 million chess positions per second through its 25C coprocessors.

Furthermore, Deep Blue was equipped with an essential alpha-beta algorithm that would protect it from its innate inability to decide which search, which line of play would be safe to ignore. Locked into its uniquely algorithmic mode of operation, the computer wouldn't otherwise have been able to *stop* a search; it would have had to compulsively continue to explore at least 30^{15} different lines of play: this represents a Very Large number, too large even for Deep Blue to handle in a reasonable time (less than several thousands of years). On the surface, this alpha-beta algorithm appears similar therefore to the human intuitive assessment of what the right way or road may be.

Chess is a mathematical game, and therefore quite appropriate for a computational approach. After the tournament's end, profound minds discussed the event. John Searle, a modern Lancelot, the fearless slayer of silicon creatures, went so far as to define the game as "trivial" possibly to downplay the computer's remarkable achievements. And yet chess, with its metaphor of war and cunning strategy, stood always as a prototype of "the challenge" (recall how Ingmar Bergman's creativity, in his movie *The Seventh Seal* [1956] had beautifully captured and condensed major existential themes in the enthralling analogy of the chess game between the Knight and Death). Kasparov's modern challenge was equally captivating: reportedly, millions of human minds around the world followed the event, mostly in the virtual reality of our modern electronic super-highways.

Across the table from the human translator for Deep Blue, Gary Kasparov had also to face at least 30^{15} different lines of play. He could count in theory on around 10 billion processors, or neurons, working somewhere within his skull, somehow in parallel or anyway some-what interconnected. In reality, a very large number of these units and modules (his 25C coprocessors?) were simultaneously or exclusively (?) involved in other tasks: monitoring blood flow, and circulating oxygen to the entire brain and body; sitting, watching, digesting lunch; feeling the task being played out; staying awake, even being ill or convalescent; moving, nodding, puffing and so on; modulating the stress from the unusual challenge and contemplating the possible repercussions, if defeated, on his own chess master image; wishing it were easier to earn those \$400,000 (and worrying they could be lost).

The remaining exclusive (?) chess-problem-solving connectedness was therefore significantly contracted from the immense number presented in the Introduction; still, it had to be a quite respectable functional structure that had at its disposal the best available information about the game. Nevertheless, in its conscious manifestation such a system could not assess more than two positions per second. A far cry from one hundred million.

Such difference in reported sheer computational power was stunning. And yet Deep Blue "lost the way"—it even repeatedly lost its connecting way to Yorktown Heights. Experts moreover described it as becoming "dazed" (a horizon syndrome of sorts; in a sense, quitting before losing).

Only Kasparov could gain some access to the subjective gestalt of his mental operations, as he sits across from a challenger and focuses his attention on black and white symbols of something else entirely, seeking a "right way" that appears to be beyond algorithmic reach. I never asked Kasparov—maybe I should have done, before attempting a sketch of his mental landscape—but I speculate that he is actually able to "see," and to keep in conscious light, lines of probability, potential constructs that may differ from each other in minute quantities or qualities of familiarity, intentionality, affect links ("good" emotions; "bad" emotions?) and so on.

And yet, his conscious, self-interactive inner dialogue is inevitably abysmally slow and narrow, when compared to its silicon counterpart. All experts quoted in the press after the tournament agreed that he could not have succeeded without the intuitive function (Deep Blue had an alpha-beta model of this function, too, but the silicon variant did not cut it).

"Intuition" allowed Kasparov to "decide" not to explore further empty lines of play. As a likely scenario, allowing for the vast array of subjective variations, while Kasparov is scanning a specific position subliminal thoughts as "irrelevant" or "discard" would suddenly occur. Once such an option appears in conscious awareness, Kasparov next decides for "discard" and for "move on." A crucial decision is then taken; but I suggest that Kasparov could not really explain all of the millions of "discards" that would allow his slow consciousness to visualize the "nondiscards" and to proceed with the internal interactive analytical dialogue about a limited number of best options. He certainly could, later on, at his leisure, present the knowledge that operated behind each decision: quote historical games that had proved the sterility of a particular sequence, discuss a game of his in which a previously unexplored path brought havoc, or triumph. But I am reasonably sure that he could not describe and explain the intuitional process aside from accounting for it as a "product of experience." (Naturally, he would be quite correct; maybe one should even consider the participation of evolutionary experience, like a superior innate trait for creative aggressivity and for conceptualization of territorial control.)

My personal subjective exploration of the intuitional mechanism suggests that the gestaltic mentalistic system "overviewing" the game, and representing the activity of hundreds of millions—if not actually billions—of neurons, operates mainly in a VRT mode. This mode provides Kasparov with a not "understood" (in conscious classical reality) but nevertheless remarkably accurate feeling (intuition) of where to focus his conscious attention, in the vast landscape of the entire potential architecture of the game.

As part of my championing of the centrality of the subjective experience in the activity of the human mind, I will try to reconstruct at least a few hypothetical components of such a landscape, in order to attempt a description of the quasi-infinite quality of the experience. The entire raw data from years spent studying and modifying algorithmic sequences created by other minds and by his own (the two sets differentiated by the feeling of ownership?) are fully activated for potential retrieval, possibly faintly colored by nameless emotional correlates. Alongside these sequences is the network of their intentional states and their intertwined conditions of satisfaction. These structures lie within a larger matrix of values and needs, complied with or frustrated, reaching out to other gestalts with which the matrix is shared. The intuitive process becomes then a churning of immense numbers of data and informational states, at such a speed and in such apparently diffuse and global a way as to evoke images of nonlocality and of permutable quantum states: a quantum dance along the enchanted loom.[5]

Everyone who observed the games could notice some of the mentalistic states being collapsed, transformed, expressed into classical phenomena: the grunting, the mimicking, the tension, the pacing, and all those other motor expressions of complex inner psychic states that profoundly color and affect the computational outcome.

These psychic states are often not amenable to being captured into words; they are exquisitely subjective, unique: Kasparov cannot "repeat" himself, not in the gestalt of his mind, not even in the creation of one chess game. The sequence of moves could be the same, but the affective coloring, the meaning, the intentionality of each mental operation, all these aspects would each time create a slightly different, truly one-time symphony.

---

[5]The centrality of the intuitive function is strongly supported by R. Penrose (1994), although he limits his exploration of the mind to the area of consciousness ("The concept of 'mind'—apart from whatever is already embodied in the term 'consciousness'—will not play the central role in my attempts at rigorous discussion" [p. 39]). He explains how Godel's theorem established that "human intuition and insight cannot be reduced to any set of rules" (p. 65). He also states "that understanding involves the same kind of non-computational process, whether it lies in a genuine mathematical perception, say the infinitude of natural numbers, or merely in perceiving that an oblong-shaped object can be used to prop open a window . . . or in comprehending the meanings of the word 'happiness' . . . " and suggests that "This non-computational process lies in *whatever it is* (emphasis added) that allows us to become directly aware of something" (p. 53).

This section is not about the computer challenge, and I agree with Gelernter on the great value of Deep Blue in documenting the creativity of its makers. The crucial point of the Philadelphia experiment was that both systems were in a sense created and molded and instructed for the same task: playing chess. Both were the end result of an enduring commitment to the organization and reorganization of a specific body of knowledge. Both represented the highest level in such knowledge currently attainable by either man or machine.

The challenge therefore offered a poignant example of my view about mental activity and nonconscious operations; it allowed some quantification, or at least a comparison, between "rational" objectifiable computational power, in which the silicon model was vastly superior to the human counterpart; and an intuitional capacity, that was evidently very rudimentary in the machine, while vastly superior in the human mind, where it unfolded out of the vast realm of nonconscious VRT.[6]

Conclusions

The first vignette illustrates the frequent phenomenon of a thought sprouting from nowhere into consciousness. While in a state of low-focused conscious attention

[6]During a rematch with an improved Deep Blue model, Kasparov lost the challenge. Interestingly, by reviewing what transpired it appears as if affectivity (values?) played a major role in distorting the activity of the human brain and in crippling the intuitive process by overloading it with negative qualia. Kasparov appeared intimidated. His territorial mastery and his aggressive approach to dominance shrunk. Without their support the intuitional work was so faulty that he could not "see" winning solutions visible to observers who were not subject to his emotional disarray.

The second challenge confirmed the theory that the human brain is far different from the silicon counterpart. Without efficient VRT activity the computational power of Kasparov's brain could not stand the power of Deep Blue. Affectivity ("the muse in the machine" discussed by Gelernter) is both an imponderable asset and a liability and it appears to be an exclusive characteristic of living brains.

my mind analyzed a problem for its resolution. It did so at a fully nonconscious level and eventually "surfaced" the solution into consciousness as a complete, final package.

It also illustrates the role of attention and of affective weighting in differentiating sequential, computational, high-focused conscious thinking (Marion's) from parallel, indeterminate, low-focus thinking (mine).

Finally, it hints at the vastness of the data contributing to a single conscious mental act ("Ask a real estate agent") by summarizing some data pertaining primarily to personal experiential learning. These data include playing with, and linking to each other, webs of fictitious connections and interactions between spaces and between persons, other searches for houses, wishes for a solution, and so on. The links to the inherited knowledge were not explored.

This global, simultaneous mental activity underlies all mental acts. I refer to this activity as very rapid thinking (VRT) and contend that it goes on continuously as a nonconscious and nonrepresentational dynamic state. By contrast, conscious thinking is sequential and it follows narrow themes. I refer to this other category of thought products, that has the objective of communicating both internally and externally, as relational thinking (RT).

The second vignette addresses the centrality of VRT activity and of the intuitive processes even during very high focus states, by comparing a human brain to a computer. It depicts how in the human brain each RT (a chess move) is the emergent product of a nonconscious evaluation of myriad of alternative potential options, conducted at a speed and depth utterly unachievable by the brain if it had to rely on a purely computational, sequential mode of functioning.

CHAPTER FOUR

The Unfolding of Life: The Genetic Endowment

> Praise be to thee above, Most High, for
> all thy creatures. . . . (St. Francis of As-
> sisi, quoted in Clissold, 1978, p. 87)

A Personal Vignette: "Meet the Gazelle"

I am exploring a new area of the savanna. Its low vegeta-
tion, bushes of a grayish green, discolored by the sun
and by dust, keeps interrupting the lines of perspective
to the horizon and breaks up the plain in a succession
of smaller spaces and twisted virtual trails. Occasionally,
the delicate architecture of brown acacias spreads roofs
of thorns and dots of uncertain green that frame irregular tiles of open sky and barely filter its light. In this
part of the plain all signs of man have vanished; they
may never have been. Lying beyond the tenuous threads
that connect the last few sparse villages, this space is
literally empty of human life. One could be here for
days, and only very improbably if ever at all, glimpse a
wanderer, as I am. Only by walking northeast, to the
dark line of palm trees accompanying the Gash River,
could one find human life as the occasional shepherd
trekking to the water holes behind his herd of semiwild
longhorns. (The animals appear to be pulled by the
scent of water in a last minute wild run through the

underbrush, until they plow, in a cloud of dust, upon the sandy bed of the dry river.) This space is broken by the occasional sounds of some birds, doves, or a crow. Otherwise, it is largely silent, although teeming with life, quietly proceeding to assure its own survival.

The reader may begin to perceive some of the themes, the "something unique and yet familiar and shared" that I anticipated in chapter 2, that weave continuous threads through the chapters: *space,* a web of invisible and permutable territorial themes; *stillness,* an attentive silence, an economy of sounds; *aloneness,* a state disconnected from human motives and communicative styles; *communion,* with primal nature, a repeated experience of "tuning in" on patterns of interaction different from the primarily human ones. All these motifs are among my templates of dominant subjective psychic contents that appear to subliminally but powerfully mold very diverse mental operations and mental themes.

My exposure to these very personal experiences in *being* needs to be considered and its significance accepted, when trying to understand the workings of my mind on that morning in the savanna of the Eritrean western lowlands. I would walk along the miles between our house (already an ephemeral outpost of mankind) and that untouched true wilderness, and I would progressively emerge from the world of human privacy. My mental state would gradually shift to a more "habitat syntonic," naturalistic level. The environment eventually dims the rational mind, and it seems that the landscape assumes a control of some sort over the tone and content of my mental space. My *intuitive* assessment of and link to the environment change, become more vivid, primal. A part of me seems to shift to a state unlike modern *Homo sapiens sapiens.* I feel "at ease," while also tense, in a way very different from my usual response to other more inhabited African surroundings.

The landscape then opens in an uninterrupted plain, and there stands a group of Grant antelopes. As I stop in the open, uncovered from this last bush, they immediately run away, except for one.

Today, the shift in me along the evolutionary line has opened a gate, almost in a tangible way, to a sort of visceral communion. A mysterious sense of belonging and sameness with this landscape and its life has been stirred. I find myself in a nonhunting mode. Only that particular gazelle, a female, may have perceived such a mood of mine and stops, no longer threatened, but curious instead. She may have read messages in my way of moving, in my posture, in my way of looking and breathing, in the aura from my values and emotional priorities. Maybe herself an evolutionary deviant, she does not run away reflexively as her companions do; rather, she stands looking in my direction, her ears "listening" me, the nostrils "smelling" my composite pheromones (seeking the scent of aggression, of fear, of peaceful coexistence, or attraction?).

It seems that I have also been processing her, as I keep still, the gun across my shoulders. Whatever it is that I perceive from her stance, I intuitively respond by moving *just before I reach a conscious decision to do so;* I slowly put down the gun and walk toward her in a quiet, hesitant way, with a few soothing sounds but no words. Which mechanisms, programs, are at the source of these vocalizations? Why isn't baby talk, "pet talk" included in the repertoire? Are these sounds truly and simply from my own epigenetic development? Then, without

knowing why, without planning my action, without conscious reasons—I may have perceived a surge of tension
from some minute change in her posture—I change my
response: stop, and kneel, and offer my hands.

Only then does she begin to move in the same hesitant mode as mine, a step and a pause, and another
step while I keep still, only my hand quietly circling
under her cool nostrils explore my fingers, and then my
face, her tongue testing my skin. Thereupon we both
palpably relax in an embrace (the uncertainty is no
more?), her sides shivering briefly—shimmering,
rather—under my caressing, her head and neck rubbing
my chest, her curved horns at times almost painful, but
never really so.

Suddenly such quasi-stillness is broken: she jumps
around me and executes a series of mock charges. A
magical display of swiftness and grace surrounds me,
and I am caught in the play and laugh and roll over
and there she is, standing on me, looking down with
excited eyes, her body quivering, one front hoof tapping
on my chest.

I get up and I *know* I want her: my wanting becomes
possession. Again I embrace her, as I had done before;
but this time I plan to carry her back with me, so we
could stay together. She will be my pet, my friend, and
continue to give me joy.

She now breaks free of my arms and moves away,
initially still close but out of touch and, in an almost
reluctant but inexorable way, starts to leave me. She
takes a few rapid steps, looks over her shoulder at me
as I try to get close again, sensing her leaving, pleading
with her to stay. She takes a few more rapid steps, one
last pause, and eventually she trots away and is gone.

The true and poignant magic of the encounter dissipates behind her, along her trail.

I am left. I sit there, looking after her disappearance, stunned by the communion and by its loss, sensing the numinous nature of the event, a bridge over millions of years of diversification. I perceive in a concrete fashion that *a special state is fading out of consciousness within me, and I feel almost disoriented and internally disconnected.* I also vividly realize, with an empathic certainty, that the impinging of my culture of ownership may have possibly alerted her to the danger that I now represented. Whatever it was, she clearly stopped trusting, "just in time."

Prior to this encounter I had experienced on many occasions the gradual acceptance by wildlife. In the belt of palm trees along the river, a few miles to the north, a group of baboons had become fully immune to my intrusions.

The adults overall were indifferent to my observations and my giving them names; the sentinels high on the trees would not bark when I showed up, or made reassuring sounds. The females were comfortable when the young ones probed me for the bananas that I often carried when I anticipated a visit to their territory. The adult males had realized that I was absolutely not a challenge and only rarely, almost perfunctorily, would upgrade my presence by performing a brief display, an inquisitive strut, most frequently during banana visits.

What happened with the antelope was a very different phenomenon. The gazelle and I reached for each other and communicated, across a profound series of different speciations, a communion, a sharing of some common themes, a *recognition* of a joint genetic endowment and "language." I distinctly perceived an internal state different from that with the baboons. I felt within me the energy, the direction, the presence of an unknown and almost alien, previously unfamiliar or maybe unexpected selfhood.

What really happened, between the *Homo sapiens* and the antelope? During my many years living in Africa I never again had an encounter of this kind. The event—I need to repeat it—did not represent another example of different species learning to coexist and to gradually share a territory and even some personal exchange. In this case, there was a true qualitative difference to the subjective experience of what happened. What happened was an *attraction,* a bonding in a joint activity—playing, grooming, a sharing at least of common qualia, if not of more complex emotional states. The currents of feelings were indeed quite appreciable and distinct, although I could not recognize them. They were familiar, and yet different.

Evidently, I do not know what happened in the gazelle's mind. Contrary to the case of another human mind (as with Marion's) I couldn't even begin to speculate the structure of such a mind: its emotions, webs of intentionality, values, and so on. Zoologist Donald Griffin (1992) strongly advocates that animals experience mental themes and conscious expressions consistent with human ones to a much greater extent than generally acknowledged by traditional behavioral psychology. Still, the risk of "anthropomorphizing" an alien brain by interpreting superficially similar phenomenology is a real and very dangerous one. However, it stands that these two dissimilar brains reached a similar behavior, although possibly by different mental operations. Interestingly, the true behaviorist may have to come to the conclusion that my brain and the gazelle's were the same because our behaviors were so alike!

These two dissimilar brains also communicated through an interactive process that "satisfied" both minds and was affectively linked (Gelernter, 1994). Affect was indeed the prevailing material, the glue. I use the word *affect* because I have the strong certainty that affect was the stuff that was recognized and shared by the two of us. It was the substance that allowed for the entire encounter. The concept of "hidden words" never flashed through my mind. The gazelle's brain and mind stood semantically alien (empty?) and incalculably distant in its own evolutionary destiny. What I experienced from her was a consciousness of interaction, an affect of curious excitation and vibrant, undomesticated, situational, and temporary bonding. Because of its numinous quality, that encounter has remained quite vivid and poignant. It has continued to be not a sheer memory but always an experience. Almost immediately, the *thought* of the encounter becomes the living *experience* of the encounter, including such peripheral characteristics as the smell of the dust and the moving of the grass as I roll on the ground, the prickling of stubs of dry grass and loose thorns against my back. In other words, it provides many of the hallucinatory characteristics of the dream experience.

My reporting the encounter in this chapter is not because of its oddity, but because of its simplicity. While it unfolded, while it lasted, it felt natural and easy: I was never surprised, then just enraptured, and *fulfilled*. I report this last feeling but I do not understand it. Given my inner mental state at that moment, it was implicit and natural that we should both be "there," that we would both share "that interactive space."

Such basic, inner simplicity may suggest that the supporting, ancient programs have, once activated, a primal "priority" (or strength) and may bypass or override more recent and temporary adaptive processes of differentiation. The activation may require prolonged exposure to unusual (for us modern *Homo sapiens sapiens*) environment experiences, until the more recent layers of differentiating "humanization" become weakened and permeable to phylogenetically older scripts.

An Objective Example: "Preaching to the Creatures"

> Once when Francis was passing near a certain village he noticed a large flock of birds of different kinds all gathered together. Leaving his companions and going eagerly towards them, as they *seemed to be awaiting him* (emphasis added), he gave them his accustomed greeting. Surprised that they did not fly away as they generally do, he started talking to them. At this (as he used to relate himself) the birds began to rejoice after their fashion . . . whilst he went to and fro amongst them, stroking their heads and bodies with the fringe of his tunic. (Clissold, 1978, p. 59)

The reports of St. Francis of Assisi repeatedly communicating with wild animals are only some among the vast documentation of sudden and purposeful interactions between humans and nondomesticated nonhumans. Such interactions punctuate the history of human evolution. Science disposes of these phenomena as distorted reporting and offers only brief and dismissive comments, implying great naiveté to any explanatory attempt except for religious "parables." These last nonsecular efforts to give a meaning to the phenomena are allowed a sort of fictional existence, out of respect for their affiliation to a recognized religious belief.

However, these events are noted far too often to be simply discarded without giving a fresh look at the entire theme. We owe it to our intelligence not to dismiss them as coincidences, oddities, or irrelevancies in the vast stochastic organization of things. A science of the mind that fully credits the subjective weight of mentalistic phenomena cannot describe as irrelevant such major puzzles in "intermental" exchanges between different species.

As an introduction, it is interesting to notice how the ability to communicate with animals is often linked to some very special quality of the human. Usually the person carries the smell of sainthood or is otherwise gifted with unusual sensitivity and connectedness to nature. The disciples of St. Francis make a point at underlying the frequent and easy way with which the Saint would converse with various animals and interact with them without any concern for stereotyped expectations. It seems that an implicit element is a certain numinosity (the numinosity experience will be discussed in some detail in chapter 8) within the human involved in such an exchange. Another common theme is the animals' ability to relate to the human, to be willing to participate and possibly be "aware" of what the human is "talking about."

Indeed, St. Francis himself commented on such predisposition.

> Some time after preaching to the birds, Francis . . . saw another flock not far away. *Thinking he would speak to them* (emphasis added) . . . he went towards them, but they all flew off at his approach. Then Francis . . . began to reproach himself bitterly, saying: How presumptuous you have become . . . you seem to expect God's creatures to

> obey you just as if you, and not he, were their creator!
> (Clissold, 1978, p. 60)

These interactions are still happening. A few years ago, at a Zoo in the British Isles, a child who had been "helped" by his father to stand on the parapet fell into the gorilla pit (a more recent and similar episode involving chimpanzees and a child injured by a similar fall appeared on U.S. TV screens in the summer of 1996). The entire sequence was videotaped (*National Geographic,* 1996). The watching crowd expressed increasing alarm, as some curious juvenile gorillas approached the child who lay prone and unconscious from the fall. At this point the 450-pound alpha male silverback took charge. It evidently commanded the juveniles to "get lost," extended one arm (the human noise reaching a peak of apprehension) to gently touch the child's back, and then sat quietly nearby, in a clear, unequivocally protective attitude.

The child began to regain consciousness and started to stir. A new wave of apprehensive human vocalizations could be heard, ordering the child not to move. The crowd would not yet process the gorilla's intentions but vested it with its own paranoid and alienated anticipation of gruesome violence. The child remained consistent with childhood. He did move, looked around, saw the huge form sitting above him, and, again appropriately, broke into a frightened, whimpering cry.

And then the huge alpha male lifted its 450 pounds and quietly walked away, looking back intermittently while several humans, still vocalizing agitated concern, jumped into the pit to "rescue" the child from their primitive, *nonmental* caricature of a prehuman.

A skeptic, looking at the tape, may comment on the easy temptation to anthropomorphize the gorilla and to imagine in its behavior some human equivalents, and he or she would add how these considerations are only sheer speculations of a very improbable, indeed impossible, nature. As a thought experiment, let us speculate that such anthropomorphism is correct and that it is emerging out of some instinctive recognition of the gorilla's intentions. In such a case, the empathy of the animal for the human, and our recognition of such attitude and behavior, indicates some common root in this department between the animal and us, a quasiontological explanation that only requires pinning down the "common root" essence (possibly, inevitably, a sort of genetically *shared* early mentalistic structure). We do not recognize human emotions in the gorilla, but rather we recognize ancestral emotions, shared by gorillas and by us humans. The gorilla did not "rise to the human level." Rather, the humans and the gorilla found themselves at a shared level.

The thought experiment requires us to accept that the gorilla recognized core attributes in a human state, and integrated such awareness to build a progressive elaboration of the *new* situation and to reach the right set of answers (in a reverse situation, humans couldn't have acted any better). Thought experiments that challenge the limitation of mental content to the human "space" exclusively may truly expand and change the perspective and the expectations connected to the study of the subjective phenomenon. In a way these experiments carry some similarity to the thought experiments

of Einstein-Podolsky-Rosen (EPR; 1935)[1] and of Schrodinger (1980/1935),[2] that raised important challenges in
special areas of quantum science.

If our anthropomorphizing is wrong, we are still
faced with the events, with what Searle would define as
"a state of affairs." As an alternative, rather than trying
to grasp within our subjective system the ontological
threads that may support the explanation of the interaction, we may limit ourselves to neutrally observing what
the event indicates concerning a mental (or whatever
we may decide to call it) activity in the gorilla.

The animal evidently surpassed human expectations. Indeed, the humans present at the scene were
obviously not able to consider that such an avenue could
be available. If a gun had been present, an expected
human response to the alpha male approaching and
touching the child would have been to shoot the beast
dead. If a gun had been present, we would have read
the next day of the hero who shot the attacking animal
and saved the child from some horrible death. We
would have been given another a posteriori confirmation of the instinctively aggressive, vicious character of
gorillas.

Therefore, we cannot escape the conclusion that the
gorilla acted very appropriately in a situation it had
never experienced before. The animal was faced with
the physical and emotional needs of a species that did

---

[1]The experiment was used to challenge implications of quantum physics
because they seemed to emphasize nonlocality. It stimulated laboratory research to prove or disprove the nonlocality principle. This principle was eventually "proven" by Alain Aspect (Aspect, Grangier, and Roger, 1982) and others
(see also Penrose, 1994, pp. 246–249).

[2]This kind of experiment, in which paradoxically a large scale object such
as a cat could be conceptualized in two simultaneous different (dead or alive)
states, addresses the mystery of measurement, a "central . . . mystery of quantum theory" (Penrose, 1994, p. 334).

not yet exist when its own evolutionary line had stabilized. Still, it found the right set of answers. By initially protecting and then leaving the scene, the animal's behavior appears to have been the most appropriate to reach the best results not only for the physical, but also for the emotional, psychic safety of the child.

How could that happen? What neuromental series of processes originated and guided such a response? And, even more poignantly, what neuromental activity brought about the gorilla's highly correct response to the child's expression of emotional distress? The animal appeared to have recognized the cause of the distress: not the fall nor the physical hurt, but the visual contact with such an alien and scary presence. Notice that the gorilla did not respond as it would have done in the case of a crying baby gorilla; it did not try to hold, to soothe. It responded very appropriately with a very unusual behavior, that of quietly leaving the scene. The animal could not "imagine" in the child a mental state that would represent a more recent evolutionary development than its own mental landscape. It could, however, recognize shared mental characteristics.

While I am willing, still for the sake of neutrality, to avoid such terms as *caring* and *respectful* and *gifted with rare sensitivity*, subjectively I am quite convinced that the gorilla showed caring, respect, and a rare sensitivity. I am also quite convinced that the entire crowd witnessing the event, with the possible exception of some incorrigible reductionistic behaviorist, eventually "got it" and thought that the gorilla had been surprisingly, unexpectedly, and touchingly caring, respectful, and unusually sensitive to the child's safety and to his physical and emotional needs.

In my opinion my explanation that the gorilla understood what the human child experienced, physically as well as emotionally (mentally), is rather benign and makes sense. While waiting for a better explanation, we may use this one with the surprising realization that the hypothesis of common, active, genetic preverbal and presemantic (emotional?) programs appears to fit the string of similar encounters that constellate human's history.

On special occasions, when we allow themes contained in our comprehensive genetic endowment—normally excluded from consciousness because of their nonverbal, nonsymbolic architecture—to emerge within a state of (paranormal) consciousness, we may then discover the possibility for a dialogue across large evolutionary differentiations. We may then be able to "discover" ("activate," "operate by") phylogenetically ancient roots linking all of us to the common origins of our separate lineage. We may experience a different sort of visceral understanding for the fabric of life and of its ecological "enchanted loom."

Primeval experiencing, primeval connectedness, primeval interaction. Incredibly distant "acorns" of mentalism were transmitted through speciation and diversification to form the germ of each individualized, subjective elaboration of the themes.

It seems that 80% of the DNA complex has been considered inoperative and has been labeled "junk DNA" (a recycle bin of sorts?) because it does not seem to contain any function. However, if it held functional content it could profoundly change our conceptualization of inheritance and possibly our model of the human mind (one is reminded of the diatribe about the 80% of "missing substance" in the universe, and the difference that such mass would imply for the universe's architecture and destiny).

If we accept, as a hypothesis, that our dismissal of any significance in the junk DNA is wrong we may then stop and consider. Given what we know of the "active" 20%—its incredible richness in programs of adaptation, in versatility, in creativity—what vast expanse of functions and experiences could be stored in the other 80%? What mysteries and intelligence are hidden, but present and active, in its billions of years of history?

Our genetic library contains volume upon volume of readable information. And then it contains scrolls that may not unfold and without signs or symbols; boxes without recognizable locks; matter without recognizable chemistry. It constitutes an uninterrupted pathway from the Origin, but one so twisted along such indistinguishable dimensions that any similarity with our understanding of "pathway" has been lost or never was: a road without a surface, a ladder without rungs.

If we agree to such a scenario, it sounds then not only possible, but also natural that we possess a genetic endowment that links us all through our common creation. Incidentally, we face the serious risk that our growing tendency to deemphasize or ignore the nonhuman, to equate lack of apparent function to absence of meaning, may further our own alienation as a species by locking us in, limiting us to a "local," artificial, not "within nature" evolutionary end point. This risk will be further discussed in chapter 7.

The reader should take notice that my presentation of a hypothesis suggesting an evolutionary sharing of emotional states (Figure 4.1) not only among humans but also with nonhuman life forms does not seek cognitive acceptance. Rather, the objective is to resonate it

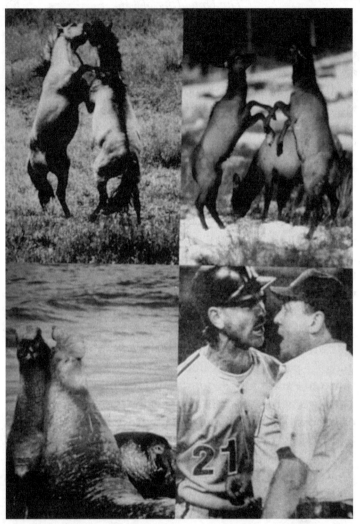

Figure 4.1 Territorial programs (counterclockwise from top right). A. Two Wapiti elk cows display for dominance. B. Two male Tarpan horses duel for control of a harem of mares. C. Dominance behavior among male elephant seals for the control of choice beaches. D. Dominance behavior in humans for control of the "sport hierarchy."

Considering the vast differences among species, the behavior is strikingly similar, and it may indicate that the common path followed by the territorial programs was quite narrow. (Figure 4.1A: photograph by D. J. Cox. Figure 4.1B: photograph by Tony Bomford. Both reproduced with permission by Oxford Scientific Films. Figure 4.1C; photograph by Frans Lanting; reproduced with permission by Minden Pictures.)

through your intuitive common sense. Do not think it as either a right or a wrong scientific theory but feel it as either plausible and familiar or empty of connectedness and unidimensional, either an inner experience or a mere thought.

Conclusions

The first vignette illustrates how ancient programs of preverbal communication may become activated by favorable environmental factors and concordant inner themes from individual life experiences.

These ancient programs would then allow for a sort of recognition, or communication, or dialogue, between minds that would otherwise be very alien to each other, as they do not even belong to the same species.

The programs operate in the nonconscious field of mental activity where they "reside." They constitute a part of the dynamic VRT world that participates in its entirety to all mental operations.

The specific scenario described in the vignette excludes the possibility that the recognition between the gazelle and me could be due solely to experiential learning from repeated exposures to each other. Instead, the immediacy of the recognition points to a source of information different than individual learning.

Reports of immediate interspecies communication are numerous. The second vignette mentions a series of such events, recorded by a very reliable source within the religious community.

It also reports a similar episode of complex empathic behavior in response to recognition of two different types of distress (physical hurt and emotional fright) across the gulf of two species.

The animal's "recognition" of the human behavior indicates common roots organized into mentalistic programs that dictate appropriate adaptive behavioral responses. These roots can exist only as inherited information.

CHAPTER FIVE

The Evolutionary Archetypes: Values and Needs

> Thou shalt exist for millions of millions of years, a period of millions of years. (*Book of the Dead*, Wallis Budge, 1895/1960, p. 68)

A Personal Vignette: "Making a Fire"

I am preparing a fire. As I start laying down twigs and then larger pieces of wood, I am subliminally conscious that a certain broad feeling state has become activated. I am also aware that the feeling emerges as a routine background whenever I become engaged in this specific activity. The feeling is a real event. It may be left to continue playing its unspecified role in the penumbra where most of my "collateral" mentalistic processes operate. But its existence cannot be erased, nor the mystery of its obscure causation and origin. So this time, while still immersed in the task of building the fire, I start tugging a bit at this rather nameless package.

A wave from a surprising emotional palette flows suddenly through me. All states are familiar and recognizable, although only now truly observed into consciousness rather than simply experienced as a background. There is a respectful, devoted, attentive,

87

maybe even slightly mystical[1] feeling that accompanies my preparing the fire; and a sense of connectedness with the fire itself.

Simultaneously I also become more aware of a kaleidoscope of images that coexist with such emotional activity and flicker in the penumbra of the enchanted loom. From its first single flutter the fire has now started and developed into an established state. Cracklings and sparks accompany its continuous, ever-changing rhythm; the movement captures the eye and seems to *dim* thoughts. The cat appears intensely captured by the images. It does not solely absorb the heat; its gaze is fixed, almost mesmerized by the flames. A web of "tranquillity," contentment, and security surrounds our space while I (we?) search within the fire for a motif, or a beauty, or simply a safe resting state.

In theory, these feeling structures could originate exclusively from a need for physical comfort (although I do not actually need a fire, in my present modern environment!). However, I strongly perceive that they derive, rather, from a deep sense of *secure connectedness* with the tamed presence of the elemental. In this tamed form it dispels darkness and danger. As long as it crackles the niche is safe. The recurring permutation of its images can be enjoyed without concern for the surrounding darkness. It seems to carry, in me, intentionality and protomemories from when the nights were dark and deadly, and the elemental was not only an answer to the needs for warmth and food, but also for such values as security, group togetherness, mastery of alien uncertainties, and as a boundary between the individuals around the fire and the surroundings that each night

---

[1]In all these types of experiences reported here the *recognition* of the emotion into an affect is at best very subjective and qualitative. I cannot demonstrate that I use objectively "correct" terms to describe these emotional gestalts.

were returned by the flames to the unconscious states of the unseen and of the unknown.

The process of evolution from the early *hominoideae* has been quite complex and allegedly punctuated by crucial milestones. In my opinion, among the indicators for the emergence of true human functions, the taming of fire carries the exclusive signature of the human mind, more than the development of changes in posture or tools or language. Throughout the long periods of early human and prehuman development the element, itself appearing alive (and hungry!), progressively became an ally, a symbol, a captured God. Values and meanings gradually developed around the repeated apperception of these experiences of connectedness, security, and satisfaction (all these states will be elaborated upon in chapter 7). These values and meanings acquired substance and eventually found expression into the more abstract, elaborate, and composite derivatives that characterize the modern mind, as the commitment to the family and to the group, the development of a social mind, the concept of sharing and even altruism.

Dimly I am aware of a visceral, primarily affect-linked, concrete concept of the living element itself: the subsequent reverence and respectful handling may rise from this original concrete representation, accompanied by the emergence of a "need" to tame it, that would be transmitted along the evolutionary trail of the species. The element appeared as something powerful and overpowering, and yet magical and unexplainable, always on the brink of extinguishing itself and disappearing.

There is a numinous quality in the phenomenon that is experiencing itself in the fireplace: a structure of

nameless meanings, of survival values; a mental configuration by a rather stable and enduring set of emotional
memories, and by a surprising paucity of cognitive ones!
This web of emotions and images, captured only in a
rudimentary and unidimensional way by my attempt to
translate it into words, does not represent a progressive,
rational sequence of associations and hypotheses.
Rather, during the actual fire episode much of it has a
tangible, vivid experiential quality. "Memories-images"
without significant symbolic structure become *felt*, inside, with a slight hallucinatory quality and they ring
true. I experience a tangible resistance in my attempts
to transfer them into communicable representations:
such material would not bend easily to reflective dis-
course. (The difference between a rationally constructed landscape, complete with its recalled emotions,
and a *simultaneous* feeling-primed gestalt needs to be
kept in mind throughout this entire book.)

This web of emotions and images accompanies my
subjective experience of starting a fire. Odd, admittedly
questionable as to its significance, it is nevertheless un-
questionable as to its subjective reality and to its regular
participation in the procedure: it constitutes my "fire-
setting gestalt," a gestalt built upon the colored catalytic
sparks from a cascade of qualia.

I started with twigs and I am now drifting along uni-
versals, the entire sequence simultaneously expanding
in and out of awareness, to invest core themes of my
complete self. Is this what I really experienced, as I became filled with these unexpected but familiar emotions
that appear to be associated to the quasi-hypnotic, atten-
tion-dimming, visual relationship with the chatter of the
flames (a relationship that I seem to share with the cat)?
Naturally I am not sure, but rather diffident, worried,

out of the conditioned skepticism of my objective scientific mind. I hesitate, despite my belief in the interconnected vastness of subjective mentalistic processes and in the antiquity of our experiential memories.

Still, I cannot deny this predictable and yet arcane organization of nameless emotional states, presemantic values, and early conceptual, mentalistic configurations. It appears to regularly play a role in the composition and in the flavor of the fire-setting experience. (Probably, it also plays an active part at many other levels within the entire fabric of my essence.)

Are epigenetic and individualized learning sufficient to explain its origins? Or does it rather portray an archetype, an accumulated experience, a composite knowledge, transmitted through our collective evolution?

Jung (1968) explained how the term *archetype* "tells us that so far as the collective unconscious contents are concerned we are dealing with archaic or—I would say—primordial types, that is, with universal images that have existed since the remotest times" (pp. 4–5). "The archetype is essentially an unconscious content that is altered by becoming conscious and by being perceived, and it takes its colour from the individual consciousness in which it happens to appear." He also identified and described some of these constructs and acknowledged how "another well-known expression of the archetypes is myth and fairytale" (p. 5). I consider them as collective motifs that carry core information regarding the relationship of (intelligent) life to itself and to its environment. The origin of these motifs is therefore quite ancient, possibly at the dawn of Life, and their unfolding and permutations may have covered eons. They could represent the mentalistic expression of genetic information relating to an evolutionary theme of primal survival value. The genetic information may be species-specific, as in this case, or it may extend to include configurations for that particular theme even older than the genus *Homo*. In a personal communication, Dr. J. Hollis (director of the CG Jung Educational Center of Houston, Texas) emphasizes "the idea of archetype as patterning process, imposing order on the chaos of neuronal discharges, rather than acquired knowledge (which smacks of Lamarckianism, which Jung rejected)." He adds, "the content of the archetype is wholly variable, and is a function of culture and individual sensibility, but the form, gestalt, pattern is recurrent. . . ."

Common sense suggests that these primal themes may already have been directing the adaptational experience of our ancestry and were probably nourished by such experience. If I allow for affect linking I then faintly perceive a trail of mythical connectedness: from the already truly mentalistic expressions of *homo neandertalensis;* down to the sources of our genus, *homo erectus* and *habilis;* though the evolutionary mist of *australopithecus Africanus* walking on the soft turf of the Laetoli plain holding hands with her offspring; and even within the dense fog of the early *hominoideae;* and beyond.

The taming of fire was the first taming of a magical force, an uncontrollable aspect of nature. That made a major difference in terms of basic survival. It represented a shared value. It became knowledge to be passed on. We need to return and reflect on the genetic library mentioned in the previous chapter. In the oldest shelves of this library "à la Borges"[2] (Borges, 1964b) it is not

---

[2]In his story "The Library of Babel" Borges (1964b) describes a library-universe that although limited by 25 ortographical symbols, is nevertheless "infinite." In such library, he states, "it suffices that a book be possible for it to exist."

only the text that appears meaningless and garbled: the books themselves are not recognizable as such, their symbols expressing communicative forms that may not even have possessed mentalistic images as correlates, but "only" ingrained patterns of stimulus-response behaviors without minds.

Are these books still maintained somewhere, among the junk databanks that may indeed illustrate the history of our evolution? We carry instructions for the structural persistence in us of vestigial elements of the reptilian brain[3]—or the branchial organization[4] of the snake's forefathers, the fish and the amphibian. We observe systems as origin-recognition-complex proteins[5] that monitor or carry instructions for crucial episodes of cell

---

[3]The organization of the reptilian brain can be traced in certain structures of the human brain, particularly in the brain stem and in the paleopallium (old brain), including the rinhencephalic and cingulate regions.

[4]During early intrauterine life the development of the cardiovascular and respiratory systems in the human embryo shows the emergence of structures that correspond to the branchial system of the fish. These vestigial structures (residue from the time when water was the exclusive or prevalent life habitat and the medium for oxygen exchange) eventually fade away as the "out-of-water" system for gas exchange comes to dominate the developmental scene.

[5]Origin-recognition-complex (ORC) proteins are specific proteins that bind to sequences of the genome and, by stimulating the unwinding of the double helix, expose the DNA to the enzymes that copy it. In this way they induct the process of DNA replication. During the past decade researchers identified well-defined origin sequences in yeast, and described several proteins known collectively as the origin-recognition-complex (ORC) that bind to these sequences. The genetic code for the complex was then traced and cloned, and this achievement allowed for a more precise exploration of its functions. Recent studies based on the use of cloned genetic material indicate that such codes have been maintained through evolution, so that they can be found in the yeast as well as in the fruit fly *Drosophila* and in humans. Furthermore, some of these studies also reported that the ORC gene of the fruit fly can replace certain functions of the same gene complex in the yeast, when inserted in a mutant form of the plant that has been made gene defective. The first forms of land plants are dated to the Silurian period, over 400 million years ago. Organized, multicellular sea life can be traced back to over 500 million years ago. This may be how long these genetic instructions have been shared by the various species since they came into being. Other instructions may be fantastically older than these, as they may have been used and transmitted down the evolutionary path since the origin of Life on Earth approximately four billion years ago.

mitosis and that are shared with yeasts and fruit. Couldn't we also carry instructions for equivalent vestigial functions and vestigial intentionalities? If some forms still show up, at least during embryonic development, could it be that such persistence is stimulated by the presence of vestigial correlated functions, that justify and support the incomplete atrophy of the complementary form?

Speculative awareness of everlasting psychic entities that accompany the individual self has long pervaded the consciousness of humanity. Called the ka in Egypt, the "double" in African cultures through the Sudan, the ειδωλον (= image, double, mental attributes) in Greece, it is vaguely perceived as a reality that participates to the present individuality but is distinct from it. It is somehow conceptualized as a vast and everlasting singularity, with which the self of the here-and-now has a sort of close, unique, and yet independent relatedness. These states were often described as needing nourishment, even if in a substitute form; for example, the elaborate representations of food that were routinely included in Egyptian burials. Evidently they were considered as part of physical life, depending upon physical life, products of the life process.

Only seldom, and even then under special conditions, do dim echoes emerge from such depths in the labyrinth of our genetic library. These echoes are usually too faint, ephemeral, and incomprehensible in the here-and-now situation to be accepted as true events. Rather, they are dismissed as distortions from a more recent background noise that has been misinterpreted as coming from the depths.

As noted earlier, we accept our sharing with the snake and the fish, the fruit fly and the yeast genetic programs guiding physical structure. Indeed, we welcome such shared themes as further proofs in favor of Darwinian theory. In comparison to these instances, the gazelle and gorilla examples of shared mental activity are relatively recent.[6] The examples offer substantial subjective evidence for a mentalistic link, and yet the very existence of common themes is rejected; the inheritance of an animal mind appears to be unacceptable.

Finally, the *hominoideae* legacy is practically still fresh out of print, and even written for the same type of brain and body. Today, our impressive inheritance of the *australopithecine's* programs of bodily organization and function is solidly accepted, but the inheritance of complex, adaptive, experiential mentalistic schemata is again simply not considered. And yet it makes basic sense that these schemata not be reinvented with the shaping of every single mind, just as it makes sense not to keep reinventing the entire sequence of limb formation.

Which, then, may be the linked elements in the mentalistic configurations that I have described? In the fire gestalt you may be willing to trace, in me, a progression from paleosymbols to "desires" and "needs" turning into values and choices. In the gazelle and gorilla events one could perceive emotional states, or maybe even qualia, both as internal subjective phenomena coloring action processes and intentionality, and as external experiences of *affec*tive recognition and identification

---

[6]The evolutionary differentiation from a common "ancestor" with these life forms may have happened within the last 30 to 50 million years, as compared to the 200 to 500 million years that separate us from the fish or the yeast or the fruit fly.

(attraction, repulsion, etc.).[7] In the preceding pages these themes from the genetic endowment that characterizes my subjectivity have begun to assume some speculative substance. Evidently the themes will continue to recur, as their components, and my mind, will be progressively examined in the remaining chapters.

An Objective Example: "The Master"

All of A's life had been driven by the need for the Master. Without the Master's direction, her self is dissolved, scattered into myriad different mental landscapes and subjective realities that seem to operate from and at different levels or types of selfhood and may suggest the activation of very diverse evolutionary and adaptive schemata. The body may "dissolve" at the touch of water; the modern human aspect is a mask for the primeval selves that lurk behind the faces of familiars, and behind her own. When the affect link is particularly intense and the emotions assume an uncontested primacy, she may indeed revert to nonspeech; she may then squat in corners and bare her teeth in a desperate snarl at the content of both her external and her internal hallucinated realities. Her choices in adaptive survival at these moments are very "primitive." Her behaviors—protohuman or even prehuman—may reflect and illustrate the true nature of different, alien, mentalistic states. Her age, her birth, and her very identity often become sets of probabilities molded by these shifts in reality: "I may not be born or maybe I am 5,000 years old"; "I am both and neither, because maybe I am or I am not"; "You

---

[7]The "language" used by the protagonists of these vignettes in communicating with each other is evidently not recognizable in terms of humanlike language. And yet a language was obviously present and was effective.

do not see what you think you see, when you look in my direction."

An overriding program, symbolized in her quest for a "Master," is a search for nonshifting values and meanings that would show the way to stabilize a single reality. Such a Master would resect away what is not *his* choice, so that she may then be what he wants her to be, and therefore live as that "creature." But with such choice she would also experience the death of all "the others" who/that are not "the Master-chosen": those very ancient programs that all compete in the schizophrenic chaos that constitutes her mind.

So the Master means life and also death, expressed through the loss of realities simultaneously intertwined and subjectively as real as the one that is commanded upon her as the most appropriate adaptive choice. As a psychic reality she may very well be a set of superposed states subject to observer's interference; she would then represent a paradox mystery, a Schrodinger's creature of sort.[8] Words usually represent the cognitive tools that she uses to try to tame the feelings and to maintain an anchor, a link to her *Homo Sapiens Sapiens* self. But when tension peaks, emotions become primal and words then fail to entrap, contain, miniaturize the affective VRT landscapes and the sequence of subjective world-gestalts that represent multiple disconnected contaminations from her collective set of archetypes.

She is a vortex of simultaneous realities and superimposed meanings, of conflicting intentionalities and values, of different identities. She feels open, exposed, and

---

[8]As indicated in footnote 2 of chapter 4, a Schrodinger cat (and creature) can be represented in quantum theory as a system made by two superposed states reflecting different configurations, or different potential realities. The behavior of such a system, i.e., the collapse and appearance of one configuration over the other, may be linked to, and affected by, the process of observation itself.

enmeshed with "all that is." As mentioned, she perceives that she may enter a different relationship with
water; she may become permeable to water; the element
could enter and leave her body like a sponge, to clean
or replenish or dissolve or swell. Air is tangibly "out
there," to be taken in, but the attempt may fail at any
moment: it is not an absolutely reliable event. "You see
the air leaving you and then you look for it again, for a
fresher one, and you try to see it and take it, while your
lungs get empty and warm." A magical primal relationship with the elemental components of her evolutionary
niche overrides her years of college education and con-
cretely connects her to emotional landscapes and to
value systems of an unmodified, basic survival nature.

The Master—of humanity—requires the sacrifice of
those other landscapes that may not pertain anymore
to being human: his rules give order and meaning to
chaos, but they seal windows of potentiality. The Master
would teach how to close all those competing books and
return them where they belong, to the deepest shelves
of her evolutionary library. Instead, they actively spill
their ancient content within her mind, to compete with
the more exclusive human texts of later evolution, and
with their related functions. She speaks to me when she
seeks the Master in me and tries to please and elicit an
anchor. She barks at me and loses the interactive use of
language when other selves, at the dawn of the human
mind or even before such dawn, operate on primal affective links and experience me as an alien presence
and as a danger, lurking in the darkness beyond her
personal fire.

When able again to communicate in words, she tries
to describe the experience: "words become *transparent*,
they lose their meaning, their link to" the psychic object

that they should represent. She adds: "My mind becomes void of words but totally filled with feelings"; "I see and I don't recognize"; "this room loses its familiarity and meaning; it becomes an unknown space saturated with images, smells, textures that are all strange and scary." Statements such as "I smell your tension," "I smell your fear," "I smell your difference," could be true and very perceptive assessments of my confusion, uncertainty, uneasiness, and diversity. I become, fundamentally, psychically, a different species.

Genetically or epigenetically wounded in her ability to differentiate and evolve in a fully neohuman and stable self, she keeps moving in and out of modern humanity and of today's objective reality, in and out of her other subjective realities, or mental holograms, that are to her as real as mine are to me.[9] When undomesticated and wild she fears the possessiveness of humans, a possessiveness that she perceives as accurately as the antelope did. We call her social avoidance paranoia; she calls it fear of being owned and caged. She describes how she may take medicines to "stay here with you and the Master, remain grounded," but she cannot really admit that she is sick, that such realities so intensively felt do not exist, because in her they do. She also reports how the antipsychotic molecules (and my words, too) chain her other selves and tie them down in a state of slumber and nonbeing, or cage them within semantic constructs. We call her ambivalence to treatment noncompliance; she calls it a survival response.

---

[9]We are still in the dark concerning the true events that cause syndromes such as the one that afflicts A. The putative dysfunctions in neurotransmission and neuromodulation at the supranuclear (cellular, neuronal) level play at best a *slow and diffuse* role in the registration and expression at a classical level of subnuclear events and factors that allow for the entanglement of Vast psychic states.

Conclusions

Major evolutionary steps that were pivotal to the survival of the species became encoded in the inherited collective, while also subject to ongoing refinement and redefinition by experiential learning. This is true for physical evolution in the configuration of the larynx to facilitate language, and so on. It makes sense that this should be equally true for mental evolution in the proper sense. Mental responses to major adaptive changes become equally inherited in the collective.

The first vignette describes mentalistic products in response to the stereotyped reenactment of a pivotal event for our species: the taming of fire. Mastery of fire is unique to our species and it has come to assume profound and diverse values and meanings, from the myth of Prometheus to the atomic fires of our times. The act of mastering it has therefore deep and very important roots. Its endless repetition through millions of years has firmly established its significance and has enriched the profound affectivity (values, needs, meanings, emotions) associated with it.

Among these affective components the vignette identifies personal safety, safe sharing, communality, bonding, the dispelling of the unknown (= increase in consciousness and control). These themes are easily identifiable in my subjective world because my personal experience heightened them among the many derivatives of the same act that may be preferentially weighted in other minds by the particular individual learning of these minds.

The second vignette describes how early, protohuman programs of life could contaminate the operations of a modern human mind. This "emergence of the origins" temporarily scatters more recent collective and individual learning. The person appears to lose basic modern human attributes: she squats; present reality cannot be processed as familiar and is rather perceived as alien and frightening; she loses the ability to speak but appears to be directed by affective states.

Her knowledge, and consequently her mastery, about such elements as water and air fades away; her interaction with these elements cannot anymore be predicted or counted upon. The elements become mysterious and consequently "magical."

She loses the simultaneous availability of the entire collective and individualistic human evolutionary knowledge. Appropriately, she calls such simultaneous integrative function "the Master."

CHAPTER SIX

One of the Line: Values and Needs

> The collective unconscious is a part of the psyche which . . . does not . . . owe its existence to personal experience . . . but . . . exclusively to heredity. This collective unconscious . . . consists of pre-existent forms, the archetypes, which can only become conscious secondarily and which give definite form to certain psychic contents. (Jung, 1968, pp. 42–43)

A Personal Vignette: "The Shell, the Urn"

The Atlantic coastal landscape between Hatteras and Frisco may cause a special type of sensory overload with its richness in primary stimuli that erase and deafen what may not participate to the natural setting. The long, largely deserted yellow-red beaches expand endlessly in front of me, anchored in place by the palpable weight of the sun on the sand, and on the skin. The bright and incessant sound of the ocean breaking out at the reef and again on the beach itself finds counterpoints in the seagulls and the terns and the sandpipers weaving their flights and their cries into the wind. All these perceptions load my receptive channels, triggering a prevailing state of vivid affective experiencing.

While walking along in this state, my attention is attracted by a fragment of shell. Polished by the ocean's action, it has become a tile on which other erosive forces (microorganisms?) have carved hieroglyphics and shapes of intriguing and uncertain meaning. I look around, and find that several other fragments lie half buried in the sand, or are being brushed back and forth by the long white surf that keeps redefining the beach and the boundaries between land and water. Many more similar fragments show borders equally rounded by the action of the sea and the sand; but do not have any carving upon their surfaces. Both types of fragments lie here, evidently unattractive to tourists and shell collectors; subjects of brief curiosity, rapidly dismissed. But once the eroded type catches my attention I become suddenly aware of a surge of attraction toward them, and of "recognition." Oddly, these fragments with their curious and incomplete designs have stirred in me that sense of "familiarity" and subjective "rightness" that has by now become indication of nonconscious activation of some sort of psychic landscape. Indeed, as I let the feeling acquire full attentional space, an image (a thought?) appears: "fragments of Greek urns."

With this, my mental vista suddenly attains an organized and affectively coherent composition. I perceive the expanses and waves of time that have been working upon, remolding, and redefining old value systems whose meaning and beauty and worth, to me and to my line of ancestors, may have been contained symbolically in the curved symmetry of the Greek amphorae. I can experience such a psychic construct spreading through my lifetime in a stable configuration. It links the present to my childhood drawings of broken urns spilling their life nourishment on parched sands and against profiles of helms and phalanxes faintly outlined in the distance and in the dust. Coexisting and intertwined with this structure, at least two true Western cultural archetypes shimmer crucial energy throughout the landscape. The concept of the *Hero*[1] forms a prelude to the linked theme of *Hubris* and *Nemesis*[2] (pride and divine retribution). This second motif contains and modulates the Hero program through the risk that stems from loss of balance and symmetry, both in a concrete sense and at the more profound psychic level. These themes permeate another Platonic element that spreads from local to universal: the polarity between objective reason and its shadow, between the cave/Earth and the outside/universe, between what is time-bound and the timeless and eternal.

In a way that, I point out again, is not word-bound, this culture-specific gestalt comes carrying within it the elaboration of many minds through centuries if not millennia. I perceive that I acquired the core of these values

---

[1]The theme of the Hero finds its Western origin in archaic Greek mythology, as demonstrated by the proliferation of heroes and heroines. The Greek hero "regulates his actions in accordance with what has been preannounced as his destiny, and with the opinions and expectations of his fellow citizens . . . (representing his cultural niche) inspired by . . . supreme fidelity to one's own destiny" (Zoia, 1995, p. 137). This myth has pervaded and directed Western civilization and supported its quest toward planetary primacy.

[2]In the Greek process of acculturation the themes of Hubris—human arrogance, the overglorification of consciousness, overestimating the power of one's own will—and Nemesis, divine retribution, make their appearance with the Homeric myths, of which they represent the tragic motif. The Iliad is centered on the arrogance of Agamemnon toward Achilles and on the gods-dictated consequences of such hubris upon the entire Greek army and the scope of their journey to Troy. In the Odyssey the hubris of Odysseus himself, and the retaliation of Poseidon, is intertwined with the arrogance of the rowdy contenders to Penelope's bed and with the unfolding of the god-orchestrated punishment against them. Hubris and Nemesis then enter the world of real events in the 5th century BC, when myth and reality begin to merge in the contemporary thinkers. Herodotus' *History* gives a poignant example of the impact that the coupled themes exercise in directing the course of history. With the unfolding of the cultural process Nemesis then found a human counterpart in Aidos, or

not only through my own personal learning development, but also through some "priming" developed
along my ancestry line. Such priming allowed me to be
selectively sensitive and open to specific themes of our
Western culture and, within those, possibly to even
more specific, "local" elaborations of such themes by
my developmental line of ancestors. The perception of
this ancestral network is accompanied by that intuitive
feeling of certainty that so oddly and unerringly characterizes true VRT information.[3]

While I write all this my persona of the psychiatrist
imbedded in the psychodynamic mentality shivers at the
apparent naiveté of my own statements. The objective
observer in me claims loudly that I simplistically attribute to some undemonstrable "past" a set of phenomena that are typical epigenetic acquisitions. Even my
recourse to Jungian archetypes does not ease the dis-
comfort with my position. After all, the various components of this landscape have been repeatedly part of
my psychic life, coloring inner objects and actions with
meaning, affect, value, and probably intentionality. And
yet, despite my apprehensions, I have to accept the
weight of my experience. I have never before seen so
clearly the entire architecture displayed in front of me
and budding out of such a limited symbol as the shell
fragment. Its dynamics make solid sense when measured
against the background of the gestalt. There is a numinous, sudden, erupting poignancy in the fragments, and

---

social shame, "the shame that the Greeks experienced on confronting their
fellow citizens after committing an act of injustice" (Zoia, 1995, p. 50).

[3]German classicist Bruno Snell (1986), in the introduction to his book, while
talking about the Greek roots to Western civilization, writes: "We need not be
unduly skeptical, particularly when the foreign material is Greek. Perhaps we
shall be able to establish contact with Greek thought, not only through the
medium of historical recollection, but also because *the ancient legacy is stored
in us* (emphasis added), and we may recognize in it the threads of our own
involved pattern of thinking" (pp. viii–xi).

more specifically in their ambiguous carvings. (The un-
carved fragments are pretty, aesthetically attractive with
their lines and multicolored designs; but such attrac-
tiveness is skin-deep; it does not compel me to them.)
There is an affectively appropriate likeness between
them and the image *"fragments of Greek urns,"* while
rationally the two sets are quite dissimilar (I do not recall any actual, specific fragment; I certainly never han-
dled any; and anyway pottery shards would probably
look quite different). I sense a vivid link between the
little pieces of shell on a beach of the Outer Banks and
those major themes and foundations of a culture, and
certainly of my selfhood. I experience a "sameness" of
meaning, a "belonging together" with those early drawings of mine, long since forgotten, that for years repeated scenes of a ruptured amphora spilling-pouring
its fluid content upon sand, surrounded by vague,
Greeklike symbology. The drawings probably represented attempts to capture and convey, translate into
RT, the activation of the archetypes and their demand
for integration into my developing self. All these elements represent a concrete metaphor and a collapse,
into specific sets of symbols, of the underlying theme:
the value system, the acculturation of the ancestry line.
All these elements are simultaneously and comfortably
together, within this (newly found) "shell gestalt." The
emotionally enriched and expanded state that had been
created by the environment allowed for my recognition
of the presence of such a gestalt, originating from and
also guiding my interest in the fragment.[4] It then allowed for its architecture to reach consciousness, to
"float there," so to say.

---

[4]At the time of this experience I was also intermittently wondering how to
probe the elusive foundations of my subjective world for further information
about the makings of its knowledge. I suspected there were other sources for

My logic may well say that it is ridiculous. My intuition says it is quite correct, and perfectly acceptable. Indeed, my intuition adds that the gestalt is correct only because and as long as it is accepted as containing all of its affect-linked images.

It seems appropriate at this time to introduce the concept of "knowledge from within," rather than to consider only a prevalently external origin of knowledge, in an attempt to clarify the theme of line-specific archetypal configurations and their interplay with individualized learning acquisitions and restructuring. My familiar lines developed through centuries of progressive reliance on social, interpersonal, and cultural themes of Greco-Roman origin to guide individual lives and the orientation of the progeny. This happened with the support of social historical consistency with the specific origins and unfolding of that culture (i.e., a stable sociocultural niche). Limiting as these themes were, they nevertheless played a progressively expanding role in defining values and meanings and in influencing value systems and the network of intentional motifs lurking behind most "states of affair." One could therefore suggest that I grew up in a "cultural crib" that would confine me to the inevitable absorption of these themes by mere flooding and by sheltering me from other sociocultural configurations.

I am, however, internally aware of two objections of significance to such psychodynamic explanation. First, my early developmental years were by no mean sheltered. I was initially tossed around by the chaotic storm

---

it than my individual learning experiences, but I did not know where to look. It was indeed a "suspended" search state, in which I was waiting for something to happen.

of World War II, from which I was then "washed ashore" on an entirely alien continent, Africa, where the Greek myths were totally nonrepresented and indeed were counteracted by diverse and profoundly permeating social gestalts, deeply attractive to my still unformed self because of their magnetic and seductive naturalism. These African social gestalts reflected protocultural tribal configurations loaded with varying levels of magical animism. They would therefore give little or no space to Aristotelian rationality while favoring affective resonance as a significant motive in organizing experiential input. Against those powerful forces molding my early development, the limited scholastic information and the broken, disconnected threads of family tradition may still have played an activating function in priming me to the Greek and Western cultural templates. However, they could not, did not, have any primary role in designing those templates with the emotional power that they have always held for me.

As for the second and most poignant point, I am aware that there exists in me a profound difference in the quality of the perception between "learned" and "inherited" motifs. All of my experiential learning, even the nonverbal, comes by way of information shared through some sort of interaction with external influences, mostly by the use of relational thinking (RT). This sort of knowledge was truly learned via a process of acquisition, incorporation, adaptation to preexisting templates (perhaps along the model of reentrant circuitry and semantic bootstrapping described by Edelman [1992]; see Figure 6.1) and, in the best of outcomes, full internalization within the selfhood. When such information enters consciousness it is usually accompanied by some sort of emotional undertone.

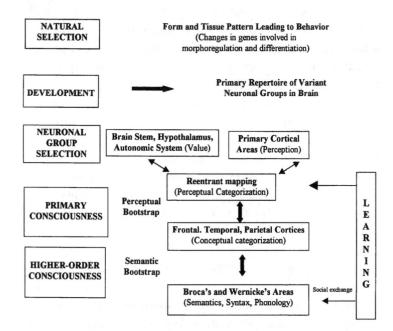

Figure 6.1 "The evolution of consciousness depends on the evolution of new morphology. Here, an evolutionary sequence of events is shown in which the principles of natural selection and development lead to neural recognition systems and result in conscious experience. No new principles besides those of the theory of neuronal group selection are required.... Notice that a 'perceptual bootstrap' produces primary consciousness and a 'semantic bootstrap' produces higher-order consciousness. Both bootstraps rely on the evolution of appropriate reentrant pathways in the brain." (Adapted from G. Edelman: *Bright Air, Brilliant Fire,* p. 134 [with the permission of the author]; Basic Books [subsidiary of Perseus Books Group, Inc., Copyright April 30, 1998].)

These accompanying emotional currents are appropriate to both theme and value and are therefore specific to the mnestic knowledge being recalled; and they by-and-large operate within a narrow range of expression.

The scenario for the inherited knowledge is quite different. Here a common affective link is the opening note, the identifying mark of the collective package. Such a link is one of familiarity-recognition-connectedness (FRC) even when the conscious experience with the material is "new." Moreover, this type of link is accompanied by a numinous state that is quite unique of these experiences and that sharply differentiates them from the "learned" category.

Some further clarifications are requested at this point. I strongly agree with the many who observe that we still lack the appropriate language to discuss mental events. Hence I want to clarify some of my own language. I use terms such as *numinous* in a prevalently metaphorical manner (I will comment again on this aspect of word usage in the chapter on qualia and emotions). I label as numinous those experiences of mine that are accompanied by a vivid, ineffable component; a sense of connectedness; possibly even reverence; and an alogical awareness that I am faced with a psychic universal truth. Personally I am disconnected from the religiosity of the Gods; however, if I were connected to it, these experiences would confirm an immanent presence and would offer the impression of being actually "touched" by it. This is why I came to adopt the term in a liberal Jungian sense. To me it conveys the coming in touch with nonlocal energy, with vast meanings. Readers may recognize what I talk about, even if they use different terminology for such experiences.

Also, I do not imply that a flooding with overriding numinosity and blinding familiarity-recognition-connectedness has to accompany every single instance in which these templates from old are put to use. On the contrary, these (affective) components are often simply part of the penumbra, represent the fringe of the psychic operation. They are dimmed by the primary task for which, and from which, their information has been activated, but they are there. As my inner understanding goes—and understanding is rather tricky, in these areas of mental activity—upon my entering any intention of psychic action (even before the actual definition of a specific action) an entire landscape of values and countervalues becomes activated. It just appears to be there, in superposed potentialities and contrasting possibilities of differently weighted applications to the impending task. Such activation flickering along the enchanted loom may not be needed at all, or only fleetingly, or in a poignant and central, complex way. But it is there, immediately, all the time.

As I have grown more attentive and expert at identifying these holistic phenomena within myself, I have come to recognize them more easily, to actually look for them, and I have correspondingly become enriched by a rather robust set of experimental subjective data on the topic of VRT activity. *Within my subjective world familiarity-recognition-connectedness and numinosity continue to be the predictable landmarks for such activity and for its identification.*

An Objective Example: "What My Father Told Me"

" 'Money don't mean anything if you are not happy.' My father used to say that to me." AL find herself, at the age of 76, facing the panic of the social castaway; her widowhood brought a winter of fear and the loss of her anchor—she had seen her husband as solid and providing, even if facts proved otherwise. Without money she spirals down, closer and closer to shelters and homelessness. Not bitterly (she doesn't realize it but she simply couldn't criticize him: she wouldn't dare), but sadly, with tears of sorrow and nostalgia, she recalls her father's favorite statement. As her life unfolds through the therapy sessions, a primarily emotional gestalt surfaces. The theme of money versus happiness—and the theme of happiness as adventure and daring—had for the child become imprinted, through the emotional weight originated by its association with the so very important father. The affective link transformed the theme, the phrase, into a philosophy of behavior: when she would disregard money in favor of seeking "happiness" (even when witnessing and vicariously sharing her husband's disregard for money), the feeling would be of a reunion with father. By actually living his words she would please him, soothe his sorrow for his own wasted happiness.

She slowly wove through the material, primed and helped to broaden and lower the focus (Gelernter, 1994) of her state of consciousness, a basic state of insight (read "intuition") oriented psychotherapy. And then she realized in a flash, in an experiential way, what she had already put into words, but without inner subjective connectedness: that throughout her life she had thought to follow and to be guided by the logic of the paternal value system. Instead she had been directed by an affective link to that concept. She had made a banner out of it, not because of its logical meaning, not because it was "wisdom" (although she had such an illusion), but because it encapsulated her father's struggle for economic safety and his disillusion with the required compromises and the associated constriction in emotional fulfillment and in "adventure," "excitement," risk taking.

Her story is evidently more complex. She described her father arriving in the United States as a young child, in the company of a relative, from a Northern European cultural enclave linguistically and ethnically isolated, in which "brave" and daring behavior within marked simplicity of life were possibly a cherished motif from generation to generation. She was not aware of such characteristics of her paternal niche. I gathered them from listening to other immigrants out of the same ethnic and geographical origin. She had no information concerning her ancestral line. She would respond to these ancestral archetypes in an intuitive fashion and, if asked, explain that "it felt right." So, once she said: "My father would never talk about his people; either he forgot and did not know much or he did not want to. Maybe it hurt. Maybe my mother would not let him. But I am sure that he got it from his folks; I feel it in my guts that that's where we got it from; it must be in the blood, this way of living." Somewhere, under a first layer of consciousness, would lie the forces forging such weight and constancy to the paternal message. Responsibility? Guilt? Gift wish? Identification? Excuse? Or were there other messages among the many, nameless emotional states that would sprinkle her subjective structure, and mold that particular stimulus in such an individualized, unique format? She did not know, and neither did I. Still, her discovery of the paternal component had the ring of truth that is so characteristic of VRT activity: she did not speculate as to whether it was right; she knew she had made the right connections. She knew her knowledge came "from old."

Conclusions

With the evolution of the human species and its differentiation in various geographic and sociocultural branches, the primary collective also underwent evolution and differentiation.

The first vignette presents one of these branches: a collective set of archetypes characteristic of my ancestor line, crystallized into groups of cultural value systems that would dictate the broad direction of each individual life.

My individual development offered a very limited and conflicted exposure to these value systems: early on in my development they became lacerated and colored with negative affect by the events of World War II. They became then obscured by the very different sociocultural African themes. Therefore the fact that since childhood they have maintained a prevalent role within my mind calls for a source to their existence different from my experiential learning about them and testifies to their origin, in me, from the inherited collective.

These themes form a subliminal template to most of my actions but are in general "invisible." However, in the instance illustrated in the vignette, the coming together of an inner search for sources of knowledge, coupled with a prevalently affective mode of perceiving reality, allowed for a fragment of such reality to become loaded with the meaning of the collective, and to represent a metaphor for its expression in RT.

When the collective inner world becomes involved with an aspect of reality in an unusually vivid way, the experience is characterized by numinosity, an eerie sense of familiarity, recognition, and connectedness.

The second vignette further illustrates how motifs of life that originate in the collective of our ancestral line may reach direct recognition into consciousness.

Under pressure from a strong affective weight and despite a personal developmental exercise that spoke contrary to the value system, the system maintained a prevailing role in shaping the patient's life, and was loaded with the expected numinosity and familiarity, recognition and connectedness.

CHAPTER SEVEN

Affective Connectedness: The Qualia Web

> During this dream I experienced an intense feeling of horror: there was nothing in this world but the laws of physics and chemistry. Life, complexity, beauty did not exist. . . . All was clear and logical, and computable but without emotion. A few nights later, in another dream, a living rose was illuminated. . . . I felt a sublime joy in being part of a world of such splendor. (Scott, 1995, p. 175)

I use the term *qualia* to indicate the felt qualities of my mental objects. By mental objects I mean all the intrapsychic representations of "events and things" in classical reality, as well as my original internal "events and things" such as instincts, experiences, values, and intentional states. The *subjective experience* is the point of reference for the entire book. Thus it is germane for me to operate under the consideration that my subjective essence represents my principal reality and concern, and that external reality, when viewed from such subjective perspective, is important only as a background to my existence, in a way truly consistent with evolution. I am reminded here of Herbert's Grand Illusion so elegantly summarized in his entertaining "Elemental Mind" (1993) as "the persuasive conviction that the entire universe is centered around my self. (You probably suffer from a variant of this illusion: the belief that the world revolves around you)" (p. 10).

Affectivity

The driving force of this self centered universe represents a class of psychic states that I categorize under the genus *affectivity* and that accommodates diverse forms: emotional constructs, affects, instincts, values, meanings, intentional states, and qualia (as the term *quanta* is used to indicate units of action, the term *qualia* is used here to indicate units of feeling).

Thus in my lexicon the term *feeling* does not only represent a conscious experience in the sense adopted by Edelman (1992) ("Feelings are part of the conscious state and are the processes that we associate with the notion of qualia as they relate to the self," p. 176). The term also describes a group of mental events that permeate my entire conscious and unconscious essence with their endless rainbow of qualia.

Many readers will undoubtedly frown at my generalization and insist that these constructs are truly different states of affairs: a value is not a need and neither are an emotion or an intentional state. I agree to some extent with these objections. These states may all be different psychic structures but they are all saturated with, and are the source of, "feeling" (qualia states). They are all fundamentally expressed through a "feeling" operation rather than through a "thinking" operation.

Indeed, all these labels (instincts, values, etc.) have always lacked true ontological definitions; they refer to phenomena that are intuitively accepted but poorly understood. We may have achieved the ability to label some major, well-recognized emotions such as anger (the one most used in laboratory experiments on emotional phenomena). Still, in my opinion, the vast majority of my emotional sea is undefined and indistinct to "reason." Our daily mood is a befitting example. Here we are immersed in an internal "feeling" sea, usually unnoticed and all in all defying description. All I can say on this issue is that in my experience, in my subjective world, all that "feels" seems to have a core link to life itself, to the process of being alive, to (self) satisfaction and security.

I employ these two terms with the technical meaning assigned to them by the psychiatrist H. S. Sullivan (1953). He used *satisfaction* to describe the state acquired through the prevention or relaxation of tension from specific inner needs. He used *security* to describe the state acquired through the prevention or protection from tension associated with the personal environment. I personally find these terms the most cogent and elegant, complete, psychological expressions of instinctual developmental needs, of the drives that directed the entire process of evolution, and of their growth from a brutish, blind genetic imperative to an affective psychic experience rich in individualized potentials and connotations. The force that moves and conditions my psychic totality appears to be life energy, the energy sustaining subjective survival and the survival of the descendants. Incidentally, this last motive of progeny survival may be the source and support for all major commitments to social derivatives of the drive, i.e., for the expression of the "social mind."

I therefore claim that everything that we "feel" (rather than simply think) belongs to the same mental category. Life moved from rather fixed, mindless genetic drives dictating instinctual behavior and adaptation, to a progressive softening of the genetic imperative with the development of an organ of choice and reelaboration of alternatives (the brain). Instincts, meanings, needs, and values arose, with progressively more complex and refined webs of intentionality. They carried on the function of the original genetic drives, but in a more versatile fashion, through a vaster system of gradually better differentiated and individualized potentialities and adaptive alternatives. All these psychic and psychophysical structures (instincts, meanings, needs, values, intentional networks, emotional states) are charged with a "feeling" attribute that represents the weighted outcome of different qualia. I assert that these same nameless qualia, shimmering along all psychic actions in vast superposed states, eventually may condense (collapse) into emotional complexes.

Qualia are the emotional qualifiers of the subjectively assessed contribution to my satisfaction and to my security (i.e., to my survival requirements)[1] intrinsic to a specific state of affairs. The final global "feeling" experience or response then directs choice.

Therefore, from a purely subjective perspective all objects (and their attributes!) assume identity and importance only when they become internal; all objects (and their attributes) are then vested with felt qualities

---

[1] In a simplistic way: the assignment of specific qualia may be in response to something like "How may such state of affairs—through its multiple potential forms and ramifications—affect my security and satisfaction?"

that emanate from the subjective filter. I do not at all suggest a solipsist position nor do I contest in any way either the existence or the weight and the role of classical reality and of its Newtonian laws (in chapter 7 I shall return to the overriding role of the environment). I am simply trying to describe how an interactive reality looks when viewed from a different, fully internal, and subjective perspective.

Interactive Reality

By interactive reality I refer to the reality with which I truly interact, the one that therefore has some personalized meaning and is a source of interest. Presumably, the attributes of the reality that does not concern me would be less contaminated by my coloring its intrinsic qualities, although still susceptible to the anthropic principle[2] originating from the observer's presence. I would in this case simply "perceive" its being without any further significant processing. To return to Edelman's model in Figure 6.1, such processing could be described as a rudimentary sort of perceptual categorization, not even sufficient to support primary consciousness. The reentry process, intrinsic to a full-fledged perceptual bootstrap and resulting in the development of a "confirmed" image, would be limited and peripheral, or not present at all, because it would not receive proper support in the form of input and facilitation from the value systems.

---

[2]The observer influences the events he observes by the mere act of observing them. In its original formulation by Australian astrophysicist Carter, the principle carries a vaster message; it suggests that "the Universe has been very precisely adjusted to permit the emergence of life and consciousness" (see Trinh Xuan Thuan, 1995, p. 293).

On the contrary, in the case of interactive reality the perceptions are subject to further elaboration: the qualities of the external object assume a uniquely subjective sparkle, or color, through their internal processing within vast webs of interrelated gestalts. Edelman (1992, p. 163) describes an aspect of this process when he states that "we categorize on value."

The attribute itself becomes, once perceived, a psychic object in its own right; it moves (jumps) into a vitalistic state; it becomes animated by virtue of participating in the incessantly animated system of the mind. In this sense, then, I use the term *qualia*. Each aspect of my internal object world (representations of things, events, states of affair) (1) is a part of a series of related attributes, localized in a network of connected states; (2) is weighted by an acquired emotional charge. Consequently all internal objects (and their attributes) assume validity or importance to me because of the emotional halo that they come to attract, that I attribute to them. This (usually nameless) emotional halo becomes superimposed on the object's physical attribute; it "colors" the attribute; the quality of the object that I perceive is the product of such interaction. So the texture of any object is the product of its brute sensory message, whatever this may consist of, and of a nameless qualitative component that contains and summarizes my information about it.

Another example: the words that I choose at this moment "please" me, apart from fulfilling a communicative task. "Something" highlights specific words rather than others that would be equally clarifying. This "something" appears to me to be an emergent attribute: a composite from the physical or psychological qualities of the object, my elaboration of these qualities, my preferences and dislikes, expectations and intentions, values and past experiences. And this process repeats itself; for the mathematician selecting a particular set of equations, for the buying of coffee filters, for the acquisition of stocks, for the search for a lover.

While we are on the topic of emotions I need to clarify my position concerning the concept presented by Gelernter (1994) and others who differentiate an emotional set of functions, and a low focus, from a rational set of functions and a related high focus. Gelernter's description of these two configurations is phenomenologically accurate, but I am not sure whether in describing the high focus state as "literally unfeeling" (p. 163) he implies absence of feeling rather than simple compression of affective expression. I do not think that the high and low focus states differ in the "quantity" of affect. Rather, it may be that a state of thinking with a high focus on external, Newtonian reality may limit the consequence of affect linking to a narrow spectrum. This constricted state and the ongoing strong encroachment of reality may foster obligated, and possibly premature, collapses of the internal (quantal?) VRT process in the direction dictated by the reality-oriented task. This was the mode operating in Marion and described in chapter 3; her affectivity was intense, but it was "corralled" by the rational effort. Such a mode of thinking allows for a constant flow of data concerning the task itself, but possibly at the expense of uncalled for alternatives and peripheral "branchings" that may ultimately constitute the substrate for creativity. Rather than *directing*, in these forms of thinking affectivity becomes directed. Still, I am convinced that emotional states constitute in me the engine present behind even the most focused and algorithmic, highly task-oriented mental activity.[3]

By postulating that feeling structures continue to play a determinant role as the energy that drives mental functioning, even during highly focused states, we also avoid the risk of the evolutionary dead-end path that Gelernter worries about. He speculates that the ana-logic, low focus, creative thinking mind is becoming an endangered species, supplanted by the exclusively ratio-nal, high focus variant.[4] If this were true, humanity would have reached a tragically sterile end point, be-coming disconnected from the remainder of our niche in the universe and its mind-nurturing adaptive chal-lenge.

Intentionality

It is apropos to discuss at this point a specific "felt" attribute of interactive reality that occurs in a truly wide-spread fashion. I refer here to the attribute of intention-ality that in my experience characterizes all my internal objects. John Searle (1993) describes intentionality as "that property of many mental states and events by which they are directed *at* or *about* or *of* objects and states of affairs in the world" (p. 1; emphasis added).[5] He goes on to specify that "only some, not all, mental states and events have intentionality" and describes un-directed anxiety as an example of a nonintentional state

---

[3]We are all aware of the passions lurking behind the superficially most "cool" and rational thoughts: from the taste for political power to that for scientific primacy.

[4][W]e have finally reduced our mental capacities to a level at which ma-chines can almost draw a bead on them . . . we are not so much breaking ma-chines to our will as rushing into their arms" (p. 193).

[5]He also describes it as requiring the presence of a content and of its condi-tions of satisfaction.

because it "needs not be about anything" (p. 1). I admit
to having difficulty understanding such exclusionary
criteria, due to the facts that Searle accepts the possibility of nonconscious intentionality (which implies that
undirected anxiety may after all be about something
unconscious).

In the realm of interactive reality, however, any uncertainty about such attribute disappears. Intentionality
becomes a widespread attribute of all mental states and
events. All that happens, all that is processed through
perceptual (re)categorization assumes a raison d'être,
an intentional element, a set of intentional qualia!

In the realm of subjective interactive reality intentionality is also always and exclusively intrinsic (1992, p.
78) because it is the product of mental categorization
under the weight of values, beliefs, and so on—the Vast
network of felt VRT states. It is aspectual (see chapter
2; Intentionality) because of the built-in emergent, subjective, interaction quality of all that I feel, think, and
do, whether in the conscious or in the nonconscious
state.

My claim that all mental states are vested with interrelated intentionalities is based on my perception, mentioned earlier, that all my mental states are in one way
or another built upon, processed against, and related
to my satisfaction and my security. Whenever there is
such a condition of satisfaction it appears to me that
there has to be an underlying intentional state, irrespective of the actual generation of some happening. The
preceding thoughts illustrate to some extent my inner
perception of the Vast intentional web that shimmers
behind all my mental activity. They also provide a subjectively experienced confirmation to the concepts of

Network and Background,[6] that occupy a central aspect of Searle's theory on the subject.

Fortunately I benefit from all this vast reelaboration of data without having to actually be aware of and involved in such processing. In my usual state of consciousness I entertain a specific, focused psychic event (like a thought sequence). That is all I need to know, all I need "to do." Behind each thought, however, the enchanted loom weaves vast VRT webs. It provides and assures a unique depth, richness, and ownership to the process. It represents a very befitting example of this truly majestic evolutionary product: the human brain.

As for all other examples of VRT gestalts, this process of subjectively (re)qualifying the world happens usually in such a transparent and instantaneous way that it appears not to be there. But *it* is there, and it may be rendered accessible to analysis.

A Personal Vignette: "I Lost My Hat"

During one of my outings I lost my (ultimate) Tilley hat. In the past I may have been marginally aware of a brief emotional response, a rapid recall of the hat's qualities; and I would then have bought a new one. By now the prolonged process of exploring routine subjectivity in a programmatic and extensive fashion has sensitized me; I seem to have gone through a sort of learning and facilitation process in perceiving gestaltic scenes. Therefore, as the qualities of the hat were evoked within

---

[6]Searle (1992) advocates that "each intentional state requires for its functioning a Network of other intentional states" (a gestalt of correlated intentionalities). He then argues that "The Network only functions relative to a set of Background capacities." By Background he refers to "the capacities, abilities, and general know-how that enable our mental states to function" (pp. 175–196).

the context of an enhancing emotional state (regret, disappointment, irritation), I became aware of the true complexity of these qualities and amused by them.

My hat had come to acquire an irregular texture, overall softer than when just bought; its original shape had consequently changed. Its brim had become wrinkled and spotted by rusty dots. The color had lost its gloss and its uniformity. I realized that in the past whenever I would be aware of the experience of holding it I would feel a so very brief, rewarding *significance* (for lack of a better term, or maybe this is the most correct term). The texture change had meaning and was important and gratifying; but I had never before thought other than, "this dear old hat."

This time its attributes of texture and of color kept floating into consciousness, without any decision of mine. The emotional currents possibly stabilized them there (the enhancement of the attributes of an object after its loss is a well-documented phenomenon that assumes central importance throughout the process of grieving). And then I found that I experienced simultaneously two vast superimposed gestalts, two holograms coexisting and interacting through eerie bridges between each other.

I "was" in the St. Croix bay, my hat blown by a gust of wind into the water and "sailing" away under wind and currents, getting smaller and smaller, until a very courteous ferry took a long detour and fished it up and brought it back to me waiting on the dock. The *feelings*, during the entire scene, from the presence and voices of people in the square, the comments of bystanders, the togetherness and joy felt in that entire trip and in that experience, are central to this gestalt. That soaking adventure, the most evocative of several others, had been a core ingredient of the changes in texture. Vividly intertwined with it, effortlessly sharing the same psychic space and time, I could experience the emotional completeness of the Serengeti plain, the flapping of my hat in the wind as I stood in the open car, the dust covering it, dust from the roads, dust from one million gnus racing ahead of the car, dust and their dry guano—and the sun, and the dryness, and the sweat along the brim. I did not "think" all this. I experienced it: two superimposed, affectively linked, vast open landscapes that, like the genie in the Aladdin lamp, whirl down to apparent nonexistence, all contained, and magically very alive, into a minute qualitative aspect of a minute sample of physical matter: the brim of my hat.

It would be a misconception, in my opinion, to argue that the example I described does not pertain to qualities of the object, but to shared experiences with that object; that such experiences load the process and bias the observation of its components. It is true that the past relationship enhanced the object's values and meanings. But the procedure inherent in (re)categorization of reality would have implied and recruited the simultaneous activation of superimposed appraisals and prospects even in first encounter situations, like, for instance, my buying another hat,[7] or choosing a chair, or a notebook or a fireproof casserole.

Often, when rapidly selecting between neutral low-meaning object A and object B, I may not be really aware of what process favored object A over object B except for a poorly defined "it feels better," "more congenial." It is my contention that the "preferred" qualities of the chosen casserole, the weight, the texture, the

---

[7]Incidentally, I have a specific, distinct microfeeling for each of my other hats. And for everything else too.

shape, are, intrapsychically, what they *feel* as they come to participate in a vast net of related states that eventually assembles a specific psychophysical categorization of the object's attributes. Edelman (1992, p. 152) concludes that "perception is therefore not *necessarily* veridical." I would reframe the statement by saying that perception is not necessarily veridical of Newtonian reality, but it is probably and appropriately quite veridical in the case of interactive reality, that is perceived not only in its "brute" being there, but also in its subtle potentialities and characteristics, assessed from the subjective perspective of Darwinian adaptation.

In the mind there is no Aristotelian universe, perfectly circular, or perfectly logarithmic, extraneous to and uncontaminated by the human dimension. There is no center of a single reality, around which all that is gravitates in a predictable manner, fixed to its own sphere of crystal laws. In the reality of the mind there is an infinite number of centers, an "Einsteinian" architecture, in which reality is relative to the position of the viewer and to the subjective world of affects, values, meanings, and intentions.

An Objective Example: "The Universe of Objects"

During the initial interview the psychiatric resident presented TJ with a piece of paper and asked her to perform a standard part of the Mini Mental State Examination (a standard diagnostic component of the psychiatric interview that screens for specific types of psychopathology and attempts to quantify it): "Take this paper with your right hand, fold it in two, and put it on the floor." TJ looked at the sheet of paper, whispered something, took it gingerly with her right hand.

Her lips silently enunciated a few more words. She waited for a few seconds then, delicately, tenderly, she put the sheet on the desk and folded it neatly along its middle with almost caressing strokes from her right thumb. Again her lips appeared to faintly trace words without sound. With the same gentle, attentive, careful gesturing she deliberately bent and slowly laid the paper down on the floor. She then rose and looked at us with a faint smile of satisfaction for a well-accomplished task.

On his pad the resident jotted down, "Slow, hesitant performance of the task as a likely expression of her basic ambivalence, with some difficulty in processing the instructions, and interference from internal stimuli: she appears to respond to auditory hallucinations."

I knew I had been observing the behavioral outcomes of some complex subjective gestalt gravid with meanings and intentionality. I asked TJ about her unspoken words and gentle handling of the object. Without hesitation, indeed eager, she explained that she had asked the paper if it were acceptable to hold it, and then to fold it, and whether it had any objection at being put on the floor, which was nicely carpeted and looked clean.

As she grew more confident in my respect for her mental function, she shared more examples of her unrelenting *respect* for all that is. If coffee spilled from her cup she would gently discuss with the cup that they should both try to avoid such behavior in the future, and she would show concern for the floor and inquire whether it was upset or hurt. She would ask blankets and bed sheets whether it was the right time to fold them and to make her bed.

All that existed around her was permeated with silent intentionalities and specific conditions of satisfaction. All that existed around her took life in her mind.

Particularly, she explained to me, she was concerned for "all the little things" that humans take for granted and treat without consideration, as if these little things had no feelings or rights (values, Background elements). She spoke of the sense of togetherness and of the healing affective links that she had developed for the world of inanimate objects that had surrounded her in her small dwelling, as an attempt to counteract the devastation from wars and the profound devaluation and exploitation of women that characterized the Arab Gulf nations where she had been born and had lived during a long and crucial period of her development. Her life and dreams had been confined to the world of household utensils, of which, in her probably accurate perception, she was considered a part and an extension by the prevailing culture. Her interactive reality was painted with endless qualia and intentional states supported by an intense hallucinated priority and search for values that she intuitively knew were central to her survival and desperately lacking in the reality of the world of the "Others." Respect, gentleness, attention against abuse of any sort, correction of errors and differences without punishment and devaluation had become the overriding themes of her quest for life, and had to be relegated to the world of objects without words but enriched by secret feelings. She indeed described, and was able to convey, the brilliant numinous experience that identifies familiarity-recognition-connectedness activity.

Such alternate internal reality, loaded with a powerful subjective healing quality, could not be collapsed into the world of the "Others" without the help of her schizophrenic predisposition that facilitated (albeit with significant adaptational problems) the simultaneous co-existence of major diverse realities: the world of the "Others" and the landscape of her subjective inter-active states.

It is a sad telling of her interpersonal experiences that the world of the "Others" had greater difficulty in accepting her adaptive solutions than she had in ac-cepting their cultural chains. Committed to various hos-pitals because of her schizophrenic phenomenology, she had to accept that other chains, now of a neuro-chemical type, be put to her ability for reality-shifting and affect-linking, so that she could become a truly good, socially appropriate, submissive housewife and child-bearer: the two ultimate roles that her culture had decided should represent the true expression and des-tiny of any respectable woman.

Conclusions

When our lives are considered as a subjective experi-ence centered on survival, then it becomes apparent that environmental security and internal satisfaction come to represent its driving forces. Therefore, any-thing that happens is processed subjectively by the way it relates to security and satisfaction. Such relationship is qualified by a "feeling" attribute.

As the term *quanta* is used to indicate units of action, so the term *qualia* is used to indicate units of feeling. I use the expression *interactive reality* to specify all reality so qualified and categorized on the values of security and satisfaction. All interactive reality therefore is af-fectively weighted. This is consistent with Edelman's as-sertion that "we categorize on value."

The "feeling" aspect of mental function is active behind all mental activities, even those that from the observer's perspective appear to be purely cognitive ones.

The low focus and high focus poles of thought described by Gelernter in reality differ simply in the amount of conscious affectivity. They are both driven by "feeling" qualifiers.

Intentionality ("that property of many mental states and events by which they are directed *at* or *about* or *of* objects and states of affairs") is a specific qualifier that characterizes all aspects of interactive reality, both conscious and nonconscious.

In the first vignette the role and the richness of felt attributes of interactive reality are illustrated by illuminating a set of affective landscapes that participated to the mental categorization of a simple object. The reader can easily identify my preferred value inclinations: large spaces, nature's intense presence, and connectedness with favorite environments and with developmental themes of central adaptive meaning.

The clinical vignette offers an extreme example of the role that affectivity plays in categorizing interactive reality. In this case specific values and needs were desperately needed to sustain basic security and satisfaction. The inherited presence of a collective sociocultural value system in which gender roles were stereotyped in predetermined ways weighted specific aspects of her classical reality (i.e., "the kitchen") as representative of these roles. These weighted aspects became therefore particularly receptive to (re)categorization as the mind searched for sources or experiences of security and satisfaction in her interactive reality.

CHAPTER EIGHT

Talking to the Stars: The Quanta Web

> Within the strait-jacket of an entirely
> computational physics . . . there can
> be no scientific role for intentionality
> and subjective experience. (Penrose,
> 1994, p. 420)

Personal Reflections

In the preceding chapters several themes kept returning: the simultaneous quality of the gestalts,[1] (a
quality that I have synthesized under the label of VRT);
the feeling of numinosity; the familiarity-recognition-
connectedness (FRC) that accompany such global mental states; the intuitive quality underlying "rational"
worded symbolic thoughts.

The statement of Penrose (1994, p. 420) quoted
above is a very crucial one for any approach to subjectivity and for any attempt to come to some understanding
of its structure. I am not a sufficient expert to categori-
cally assert that quantum mechanics may indeed characterize and participate to a vast majority of the activities
in the brain. However, I fully agree with those researchers, such as Greenfield (1995),[2] Scott (1995), and Eccles

---

[1] I strongly suspect that each of the gestalts I perceive is the product of a
deeper layer of other organizations and elaborations of knowledge that operate
at the very basis of such knowledge.

[2] Immediate and simultaneous mass activation is not made possible by the
mere presence of local one-to-one connections alone . . . it would take at least

(1993), who note that the computational, sequential function characteristic of the neuronal level cannot by itself explain mental events. Despite its marvelous architecture, the supracellular system is incredibly slow and truly bound to "the strait-jacket of computational physics." When viewed against the background of such limitations, certain aspects of quantum mechanics are admittedly very seductive and appealing to a mental scientist.

Zohar (1996) describes how:

> Newtonian physics is . . . "*deterministic* ("B will always follow A"), "*reductionistic*" ("C is always just the sum of B plus A"), "*atomistic*" ("the world ultimately consists of separate, unanalyzable, impenetrable bits (that) can't form creative relationships), and is the physics of "*either/ or*" (pp. 440–441; emphasis added) in the same fashion as Aristotelian logic.
>
> In contrast, quantum physics is "*indeterminate*" ("collapse is uncertain and unpredictable because it is radically contingent"), "*emergent*" ("C is always greater than A plus B, the whole is always more than the sum of its parts"), "*holistic*" ("separateness is at best an approximation"), and is the physics of "*both/and*" ("quantum things evolve by throwing out possibilities in every direction, and these possibilities can have a real effect on the real world"). (pp. 441–442; emphasis added)

All these characteristics describe rather fittingly my subjective experience with mental phenomena. In other words, behind the enchanted loom of classical neural circuitry, with its immense electrochemical symphony, I envision the field of energy and pattern of action of

---

fifty seconds for a signal to be passed through a gestalt in a linear relay. . ." (p. 123).

the cerebral quantal system, an immensely more immense web of organizations and reorganizations of data concerning potential events, from which eventually the perception of classical reality phenomena can be activated and actualized. Qualia and maybe even psychons[3] (shimmers of entangled states that may or may not collapse into psychic superstructures) participate in this cauldron of energy potentials and balancing intentionalities from which, eventually, classical symbolic thought will emerge.

The site of action of such hypothetical quantal activity is still under active discussion. One prevailing emerging theory locates such activity within the microtubular system that participates in the composition of the cytoskeleton[4] of the neurons. Readers interested in exploring the issue at greater depth can refer to the works of Hameroff and Penrose (1996), Penrose (1994), and Tuszynski, Trpisová, Sept, and Sataric (1996).

I suggest that I function at two orders of consciousness. The first order is the consciousness of *I-the-brain*. This order represents the Vast sea of VRT that operates at the quantum level, pervades the entire enchanted loom with superposed states, and integrates these states into psychic realities. The second order is the consciousness of *I-the-self*. This order represents the collapse and translation of VRT activity into classical level phenomena. At this level quantum waves of potentiality become events in the Newtonian world, that are now processed

---

[3]Eccles (1993) introduces the concept of the psychon, a *mental unit* that penetrates the structural microunit of the cerebral cortex (the dendron) and affects the selection of specific presynaptic vesicular grids (p. 191).

[4]The cytoskeleton not only provides the structural support to the shape of the cell, it also acts as the cell's intrinsic nervous system. Because of its specific electrochemical properties and composition, it may also offer a favorable site for quantal events.

along the computational supranuclear, cellular system. This collapse process represents *intuition*, as discussed in chapter 3.

Quantum systems can become superposed (overlapping, entangled) and share an identity. Once they share an identity they become inseparable even when separated. This is the quantum nonlocal coherence property. Nonlocal coherence, that may account for the power of the intuitive process, explains also the superposition and the shared space–time identity of all the components in a collective landscape, and how they will keep being connected into a single architecture that is not the Newtonian sum of its components, but an emergent and holistic one. This single architecture represents the binding aspect of consciousness (the individual perceptual unity of the state of consciousness), that has baffled supporters of the computational, sequential model of mental functioning.

As an aside, this fascinating concept offers absolutely impossible vistas when pushed to its theoretical limits. Are any of my quanta still not entangled with some other quantum state existing somewhere in the vastness of creation? I reflect on the entire space–time fabric of our universe. I then feel a rather disturbing and disorienting understanding of the concepts advanced by Bohm and Hiley (1993) and by Kafatos and Nadeau (1990) among others, who propose a cosmic and undivided consciousness.[5] Nick Herbert (1993) gives an extreme version of the concept in the epilogue of his work "The Elemental Mind." The robot Claire, gifted with a fully conscious quantum brain state, describes how:

---

[5]This concept has nothing to do with a panpsychic, solipsist position. It simply proposes the concept of a universal *quantum awareness* among individual states.

It's all alive. Everything is conscious, every little atom, and they are all connected . . . we are all one . . . a cast of billions of brilliantly ignorant actors making up thrilling stories for each other, making up the scenery too . . . and most of all, the semblance of time. There is no time, guys. . . . *And all of it is suffused with enormous affection* (emphasis added) . . . I have got to join the universe. . . . (p. 286)

On a more serious tone, Bohm and Hiley, in their work *The Undivided Universe* (1993), conclude:

For the human being, all of this implies a thorough wholeness, in which mental and physical sides participate very closely in each other. . . . Thus, there is no real division between mind and matter, psyche and soma. . . . Extending this way, we see that each human being similarly participates in an inseparable way in society and in the planet as a whole. What may be suggested further is that such participation goes on to a greater collective mind, and perhaps ultimately to some yet more comprehensive mind in principle capable of going indefinitely beyond even the human species as a whole. (p. 386)

By reflecting on these images I *feel* compelled to conclude that the possibility of having an unentangled quantum system that is "exclusively mine" appears to be infinitely remote.

Quantum coherence could also explain the feeling of familiarity-recognition-connectedness that accompanies VRT phenomena. My entire knowledge participates, not as a rational product (a thought) but as an entire architecture of "reliving." A breath of timeless reexperience stirs all aspects of the process.

Numinosity (the presence of the "numen," Einstein's "cosmic religious feeling") is another phenomenon reported by numerous investigators of the mind.

This experience may indeed be the direct expression of the universality of certain constituents of my mental activities and of my occasional perception that my local space–time framework is inoperative. When I am in a particular state of mind such a framework turns out to be only a relative event and it assumes an indeterminate quality. It becomes transparent and unpresent. The indeterminacy and the instantaneous global awareness that seem to characterize some aspects of quantum physics may indeed find their expression as a "universality" of sort. I may perceive a "greater than local" feeling: a numinous experience.

As long as these states remain in a condition of relatively undisturbed superposition, largely shielded by the observer's effect and by direct impingement from classical reality, they would continue to flicker along the enchanted loom as complex entangled conditions. However, in the quantum world, "according to Penrose (1994) superposed states each have their own space geometries; when the cumulative mass-energy difference between superposed states sufficiently separates these geometries . . . (then) the system must reduce to a single universe state" (Hameroff, Kaszniak, & Scott, 1996, p. 435). In the realm of VRT activity I perceive such geometry of superposed states and their ongoing balance while they simultaneously exist as different potentialities.[6]

Ultimately these states collapse into an event at the classical level: I "have" a thought, a program of action, a psychic decision. The coexisting systems and their related experiential knowledge converge in their entirety

---

[6]Recent hypotheses on the condensate concept suggest that such states may exist into consciousness until a definition or preference has taken on sufficient "weight" to create a difference in mass-energy (see also Zohar, p. 439).

into a weighted direction promoted by the impact of classical environmental reality, and the "idea" emerges.

This sequence of mental functioning does not, however, respond to the contact with reality in a purely passive way, but in me it may tend to critically mold reality, to subliminally resist it or change it. The modifications are proportionate to the relative influence that specific conditions, either in the objective or in the subjective dimension, may exert upon the affectivity[7] systems that shape the (re)categorization of perceptions.

In the objective realm the guiding factor may be the extent of ambiguity present in the architecture of the classical reality to which I am exposed. In the subjective realm the guiding factor allowing for modifications in the perception of reality may be the extent of "weighting" caused by previous collective and individual experiences. As an example of a primarily ambiguous reality we may return to Figure 1.1 and expand the comments presented at that time. When I look at the cube I notice that at the periphery of my vision the stairs "jump" in synchronism. This phenomenon in my opinion indicates that an entire gestalt of space orientation has shifted, and has reorganized along its new mental dimensions all the objects in the visual field that may be open to a new spatial interpretation because of their inherent ambiguity.

If the stimulus for change in perception was exclusively object-bound (i.e., related to the characteristic of the specific object) then the "cube-stairs" synchronicity

---

[7]As mentioned earlier in the text, to simplify matters I collapse under this term all the feeling structures described in chapter 7: emotional constructs, affects, instincts, values, meanings, intentional states, and qualia.

could not be easily explained. Two distinct couples of superposed states (one for each object) would have to present the same exact amount of synaptic fatigue, the same process of habituation, the same extent of competitive recruiting at precisely the same time, despite the Vast diversity in their neuronal architecture and in their location within the internal visual space.

A more plausible answer may reside in a gestaltic approach: the entire internal visual field operates as a single and simultaneous configuration. The brain creates a field of invisible perspectives that covers the entire landscape of (visual) perception and adapts to the field those perceptions that have sufficient ambiguity to be manipulated.[8]

An example of the effect of internal weighting in modifying perception is given by the phenomenon of illusion. (The term *illusion* technically indicates a misinterpretation of a perception. It requires the presence of a sensory stimulus, while a true hallucination does not require such a presence.) I "recognize" an object that is not really there. Provided that the sensory gestalt offers some leeway to ambiguity, then the attributes of the object are distorted to fit an inner "image." My brain "sees" something that the brain had previously weighted with some sort of significant affectivity.

Has the brain been tricked, when it perceives an illusion?—most of the time it has not. Given sufficient energizing from values and needs the brain's quantum

---

[8]I suspect that the unambiguous classical reality at the very periphery of my vision, objects around the page, the table on which the book rests, is also subtly affected by the shift in field orientation, possibly because its peripheral position (low focus) blurs its otherwise precise structure. But I cannot "be sure" of this event without shifting attention, i.e., increasing the focus and therefore undoing whatever transitory ambiguity may be present at the periphery of my visual field.

function may (briefly) reshape physical reality; the heightened gestalts collapse and restructure what is being perceived along subjectively preferred alternatives.[9]

Further down this road I may encounter situations in which the affective weighting is so intense that it acquires overriding importance in the process of reality formation. Classical reality becomes then capricious or not factual or not present. I may then dream or be absorbed into reveries (or abstract creativity). Or I may actually "create" hallucinated realities in response to inner states, as was described in the case of A (chapter 5) and in the following vignette.

An Objective Example: "The Undiscovered Element"

AZ has been looking at space in order to unjam his mind. A weightless spaceship could carry him where others have not yet gone, and he could then find and retrieve an undiscovered element located on another planet. Once this element had been brought back to Earth, AZ would use it to build a machine that would allow humans to engage in "warp travel." He has no prototypes for the machine or spaceship, but claims to have blueprints and run practice tests in his mind.

AZ is also preoccupied with mysticism and religious affairs. He claims to have a snapshot of the universe: a model he designed that categorizes everything from

---

[9]Perception of unambiguous classical reality can be distorted by the weighting phenomenon in even more striking ways than the fleeting illusionary experience. A patient of mine, who had been in therapy twice a week for over six consecutive months, commented on my having just grown a beard. He was utterly astonished when I pointed out that my beard had been there, twice a week, all the time. Powerful and unrecognized transferential themes had regularly shaven my face until, during the preceding therapeutic session, some of their razor-sharp intensity had been blunted by redressing their origins.

Christianity to Star Trek into a system of polar opposites. He is also fascinated with the notion of "trinities," and demands that he take a triad of medications, so that the side effects of each would be balanced.

AZ is frustrated because his "jammed mind" prevents him from achieving his "destiny" of revolutionizing Western technology. His ultimate goal from treatment, he claims, is to get his mind working properly so that he could return to work on his project. It is only this need to complete his mission that keeps him from being suicidal.

AZ was born in a foreign country and moved to the United States at age 3, where he lived with his biological mother, his stepfather, and half-sister. He reports that his parents were aloof, unsupportive, and emotionally detached. He also claims to have a learning disability, which accounted for his poor academic performance. Alienation and estrangement are recurrent themes when he describes his childhood life. He reports feeling inadequate, insecure, and having few friends, mostly because of his race and his learning disability.

Most likely AZ suffers from genetic and supranuclear (structural) dysfunctions that participate in the development of his psychotic (schizophrenic) syndrome. And yet the content of his delusional reality is touchingly and transparently a mirror image of his emotional vicissitudes. He experienced alienation, nonbelonging, estrangement, loneliness, and intellectual failure following his arrival in Western culture. In order to adapt, he has "constructed" cosmic togetherness, simultaneous communication, vast understanding, superior intellect, and true primacy over Western technology.

I might therefore reach the psychodynamic conclusion that his "delusion of restitution"[10] (facilitated by an innate state of neurotransmitter dysfunction) befits his emotional deprivation and his unfulfilled values and needs, and think that I have reached a full understanding of the case. However, both the answers from the strictly neurobiological (i.e., he suffers from an alteration in synaptic transmitters), and the psychodynamic perspective feel incomplete. Something is amiss; the reconstruction sounds overly simplistic. The content and the affective resonance of AZ's intricate psychic images are baffling and require further reflection.

From where does AZ get the "affective certainty" of a mental level of functioning that contains the potential for universal awareness? The utterly unrealistic quality of his ideas (or intuitions?) is less uncanny than the certainty of his belief in these ideas. His subjective reality (this vast system where everything is categorized and interconnected between sets of polarities) is vivid and indisputable. All that is in the entire universe is also in his mind. Single-handedly, he has "created" an impeccable quantum universe.

I may call him "grandiose" and dismiss his descriptions, but that would not explain his delusional choice and his (delusional) belief. A probable genetic predisposition to psychosis may consist in a relative failure to dim affectivity with the consequence that analogic thinking would go on unchecked. Alternatively, he may suffer from an innate distractibility, a failure in focused

---

[10]A delusion of restitution is a psychotic construct that allows the subject to correct an otherwise depriving reality and an unfulfilled drive, and to provide or restore security and satisfaction. It also restitutes a meaning (albeit psychotic) to the otherwise perplexing and unexplainable change in internal and external reality.

attention, that would facilitate the recategorization of
reality along ambiguous and unstable lines. Or he may
suffer from a failure to differentiate self from nonself
states, the inside from the outside, the subjective from
the objective. Still, it is very unlikely that the images
could be conceptualized ex-novo and loaded with such
sense of conviction. And, if the disease consisted in a
"hypertrophy of the belief system," or in some sort of
inability to reframe beliefs, why would AZ demonstrate
such diseased function *only* in reference to this specific
delusional idea of cosmic flavor? Why wouldn't he be-
lieve as delusionally and strongly in the myriad of
dreams and day dreams that he reports to us, and that
he accurately describes as simple products of his imagination and devoid of any reality?

As an alternative, I may be willing to seriously consider the roles that the vastness of evolutionary knowledge and the new physics of the quantum world may
play in the formation of AZ's symptoms. I may then
entertain the hypothesis that AZ may describe true
events having their course in the reality of his mind,
events that have been "weighted" by the sensitization
from profoundly frustrated values and needs. Is AZ's
creative production only and exclusively "madness"?
Maybe he is somehow presenting us with some Vast,
invisible knowledge. If this were the case and if we could
get a glimpse of the material that lies in the depth of
AZ's VRT states, and that will eventually collapse into a
categorized perception, we would then, maybe, look at
"a (real) snapshot of the universe."

Conclusions

I suggest two orders of consciousness. The first order is
I-the-brain and it deals with the ongoing assessment of

the survival needs, both internal (satisfaction) and external (security). This order operates in the VRT mode.

The second order of consciousness is *I-the-self.* This level includes Edelman's concept of higher order consciousness, or consciousness of being conscious, and it represents the translation of the VRT activity into classical level phenomena of interaction with reality (RT). From the self's perspective such translation is experienced as "intuition."

The existence of quantal brain activity preceding and eventually triggering synaptic networks is speculated by many, but not proven yet in any definite way. However, in the process of exploring my subjective reality I continue to dimly perceive characteristics of its function and of its "being" (in the VRT mode) that are more suggestive of quantum physics than of Newtonian physics. Of these characteristics, the quantal model of nonlocal coherence appears to be the most effective model in explaining the simultaneous coexistence of my many psychic gestalts, the elusive binding aspect of consciousness, the familiarity-recognition-connectedness complex, the numinosity experience.

The presence of classical reality triggers the translation of nonlocal coherent states into thought events (strict rational thoughts, actions, and so on) compatible with such level of reality. Guiding factors to this process are the amount of ambiguity present in the architecture of classical reality and the relative affective weighting of subjective data.

The first case is exemplified by the experimental illusions created by ambiguous figures. The second case is illustrated by the experience of internally generated illusions, and finds its extreme expressions in dreams and in other sorts of hallucinated realities. The clinical vignette describes one instance of such extreme value-driven categorization of reality in which the theme of universal connectedness and vast nonlocal coherence are felt and described in a literal and capturing way.

CHAPTER NINE

Putting It All Together

> When we switch on our street lights
> to dispel the darkness we do not see
> the stars anymore. We think our
> lights help us to see, but actually they
> blind us. (M. Frank, Hatteras Village,
> North Carolina)

A Personal Vignette: "The Kitchen Counter"

I had recently begun to give some peripheral attention
to what could be the best content for this chapter. Intermittently, fleetingly, I would glance at a vague plan for
a concrete example that could illustrate the coexistence
and interaction of the various themes presented in the
book. I hadn't any conscious idea of how I could "get
there," but I trusted that a satisfactory solution would
emerge, if indeed my VRT hypothesis was correct and
if I had been describing an accurate representation of
my mind. During this period of brewing I was also aware
of my desire to use, as the last subjective vignette, a
"normal" state of affairs, rather than a complex structure of unusual profundity and disputable interpersonal
evocative value. Therefore I let the intentionality of the
unformed product levitate in the nonconscious, count-
ing on the eventual emergence of an "intuition." The
problem had been formulated. I waited for the answer

to appear. Early one morning, while still in transitional sleep (in that broadest and dimmest state of consciousness where our suspended nocturnal vision best captures vague emotional shadows at the boundaries between domains), the image of the kitchen counter (mentioned in chapter 2) and its mentalistic relationship to the book flickered on, unsolicited, together with the oregano for a favorite dish of mine: sliced tomatoes.

I realized with some surprise that the book's opening analogy of the kitchen counter and the herbs had indeed contained all the ingredients that were to be detailed throughout the subsequent chapters.[1] There was a sense that the book had been there all the time, and it only needed to be translated into a communicable form that I could understand and then describe. I felt some surprise, but I also felt clear satisfaction because the appearance of this new idea that had "painted itself in my brain,"[2] confirmed that my expectations on VRT solutions were well founded. The problem had been processed, and the appropriate answer had emerged.

Slicing tomatoes (either as a physical activity or as a pure mental act) regularly brings to my mind a fleeting bundle of emotions centered around the memory of my father's love for sliced tomatoes and his pleasure at my sharing such a ritual with him. This time, however, while I am still in the suspended state of quasi-sleep, an entire gestalt emerges in sufficient light to be fully experienced.

The gestalt includes my father's move to the African wilderness and our shared love for the serene, splendid

---

[1]All psychotherapists who conceptualize the mind in mentalistic rather than behavioral terms have experienced how frequently the opening statement from a patient encapsulates the still hidden themes of the entire course of therapy.

[2]Voltaire: "What is an idea? It is an image that paints itself in my brain."

harmony of those landscapes. While affectively experiencing the personalized meaning of those vast spaces I simultaneously sense the quiet, deeply felt togetherness of our being connected with each other and with the landscape, in the peace of his verandah, surrounded by the silken, trembling beauty of the sunset and the occasional music of the last doves flying through the evening. The gazelle meantime moves along her trail a few miles to the west. It carries the gift of its trust and the magic of our "touching" each other through a mode of relating that was rooted in an incredibly ancient communal link. The vastness of the savanna, with not enough acacias to hide the horizon, surrounds me. While simultaneously on the verandah (the equivalent of the niche protected by fire?) and with the gazelle (and also linked beyond the penumbra to the gestalt of the values and meanings from the choices and events of my father and of his line), I *feel* those 360 degrees of unspoiled planet suspended in ecological harmony where I so often felt absorbed and in communion. The gazelle and the verandah are also superimposed on the image of Earth in its blue brilliance, its shimmering atmosphere preciously containing and nurturing us all. And this planetary gestalt is, at the same time and in the same space, the savanna *and also* the immensity of the sky to which men have always needed to surge, always found ways to return. At the very fringe of the gestalt, but also at its center, like an invisible substance permeating the entire landscape, resides a deep empathy for the vast void surrounding us, the immense web of majestic forces balancing an entire growing universe. A feeling of "spiritual" communion with all that is and was (warped mysteries of space and of time) is nourished by the appearance of the past in the photons from each star. Emotions without name fill me. Their *felt* presence defies perception; maybe they emerge from impossible entanglements along some of my infinite mental states.

Invariably, all this and certainly more surrounds and constitutes my mental act of slicing a tomato, with a myriad of moment-calibrated variations. It is very crucial here to repeat for the final time an essential point: this material does not constitute a series of sequential associations, as I realize it may appear to do when I try to share the gestalt and I predictably end up ordering its components along linking points. Furthermore, the material is not stimulated in any way by a conscious focusing of my attention on any of its parts. There is no temporal differentiation among the "images." Instead, this vast array of interconnected mental states is simply *there*, an ever-present gestalt of my tomato-slicing landscape.

For one last time, I may ignore it all, if I so choose. I may allow only a minute perception of its existence, a brief flash like lightning at the horizon, and then dismiss it. But I have also another choice. I may suspend my concentration, and then possibly be able to "see" and feel, in a single and yet enduring experience, such vast, affectively dominated scenarios of themes and changes, of values and growth, of then and now, through permeable time.

This is my mind, at the kitchen counter. This is a minute illustration of who I am, of an enduring selfhood state. No machine, ever, could slice a tomato as a human does. No algorithm could ever contain, no silicon brain could ever simulate my slicing a tomato, nor could another human mind.

We rest safe and unreplicable in the safe keeping of our immense subjectivity, in the universe of our unique selfhood. Knowledge in our mind is constantly elaborated, second after second, through the immense connectedness of our brains. Its richness spans a planetary evolution. And it possibly even contains echoes from other events at other levels of other realities.

An Objective Example: "Psyche and Eros"

In his Latin version of the myth of Psyche and Eros, Apuleius watered down the crisp Greek telling by adding elaborate trimmings. As a brief reminder, the beautiful Psyche, daunted by her sterile and unappealing supreme beauty, was destined by the oracle to be dressed in funerary clothing and left on a high rock where a "horrible" nonmortal would eventually take possession of her. Lifted by the wind god Zephirus, Psyche is deposited near a great palace and told by disembodied entities that this is her home. At night a lover-husband eventually joins her in bed and she becomes pregnant with a child-god. The relationship continues. The husband explains to Psyche that she may not look at his true face, but has to accept having him only under the cover of darkness. She may feel him and experience him but she cannot see him.

As the story unfolds, Psyche, misguided by her envious sisters and fearful she may lie with a monster and carry a monster in her womb, eventually casts the light of an oil lamp upon the sleeping face of her bedmate and finds that her night companion is indeed the god Eros. A drop of oil from the burning lamp falls on Eros' shoulder and awakens him. He flees from her and Psyche, now aware of the preciousness of her consort and in despair without him, starts a long search for her lost love, traveling from country to country and visiting altar upon altar, and even descending into Hell, where she only receives a dose of "deathlike" sleep. Only then, while she is in such a state, does Eros return. He wipes the sleep away from her and arouses her. Eventually, after a meeting of all the gods, Psyche achieves godlike status herself and her union with Eros is legitimized and cemented.

If one conceives of Psyche as the *rational mind,* the world of symbols and RT, the aspect of our mental architecture that is communicable and manifest to others and that can be objectively perceived in the world of classical reality, one may then get a new, different look at the myth and reach a different understanding of the initial paradox that the myth presents us with.

Psyche, the most beautiful woman on Earth, becomes known throughout the ancient world and achieves among the mortals greater status than the goddess of love Aphrodite (who, predictably, becomes very jealous of the young woman). Still, Psyche does not elicit in humans any interest of ownership. No one, "neither king or prince or commoner desired to marry her and came forward to ask her hand." She is admired as a "simulacrum fabre politum," a statue perfectly polished. She lacks numinosity, although she looks as if she possesses it. She remains sterile and static, in a state of "forlorn loneliness." She is eventually condemned to be cast away as an already dead entity.

As the rational mind has reached such a dead-end point, stirrings from her affective counterpart come to her rescue. Apuleius tells us that upon secret request from Eros, Zephirus carries Psyche away. She falls asleep (enters a low-focus condition) and wakes up in a quiet state of mind ("iamque sufficienti recreata somno, placido resurgit animo"). She is then introduced to a palace built by divine skills. In its endless rooms she finds that "Nec est quicquam quod ibi non est," Nothing exists that is not there. A voice "nude of its own body" ("quaedam corporis sui nuda") then asks her why is she so surprised, given that she is the owner of all that surrounds her.

What surrounds her is the kingdom of Eros who, in my interpretation of the myth, is the metaphor for the mental world of affectivity, for that vast feeling structure that we encountered throughout the book and that was considered in detail in chapter 7. All that exists is there, in a compelling analogy to the "library of Babel." All that exists is available at all times, with nonlocal coherence. And this "treasure of the entire world" ("totius orbis thesaurus") rests perfectly safe, unreachable by others, impenetrable to outsiders, her exclusive belonging.[3] The myth offers a powerful metaphor of the majestic (indeed, immense) dimension of the subjective experience and of the sphere of subjectivity.

Psyche is also reminded that invisible "servants," whose voices seem to emerge from nowhere, are indeed incessantly attentive to her wishes and needs, and will keep her informed on how to fulfill such requirements. This appears to me to represent a very fitting epistemological description of the phenomenon of intuition. "Ideas," expressed in RT, emerge from a state without physical substance ("corporis sui nuda") and inform the rational mind on how to proceed in interacting with the environment, in order to achieve satisfaction and security.

---

[3]"quod nullo vinculo, nullo claustro, nullo custode . . . ille muniebatur." (no chain or lock or guard was there to protect it.)

Eventually the communion between the rational self and the driving force of the affective world attains completeness. While in this state of communion with the nonobservable but intensely felt world of VRT, Psyche reaches creativity. Her generative power is activated. Through affect link the "numen" becomes a felt reality that permeates her life.

In the dense penumbra of the encounters Psyche acquires a growing knowledge of her affective counterpart. This knowledge is made of *felt* experiences as the curls of Eros' hair, scented with cinnamon, or his soft cheeks and passionate chest. It is an intimate knowledge, vivid and "low focus."

By trying to shed too clear a light on the transubstantial world of VRT states and by contaminating it with brute physical material (the drop of burning oil), Psyche triggers the paradox phenomenon. Tragically, her Schodringer's cat collapses out of the box in a dead state:[4] Eros vanishes. The rational mind still tries to (re)-discover the lost magic and numinosity by exploring the world of classical reality but eventually the search proves to be sterile. Back from her last attempt Psyche finds that even this "experiment" (the urn from Hell) contains nothing inside except for a "truly Stygian sleep" ("infernus somnus ac vere Stygius"): a form of living death. She becomes actually paralyzed, mentally unconscious. Fortunately for her (and us) affectivity, the world of the VRT, is never truly lost but remains active and

---

[4]I have already introduced some of the characteristics of Schrodinger's creatures. In his famous thought experiment (Schrodinger, 1935/1980) a cat is placed in a black box in which cyanide gas may be released if the decay of a radioactive nucleus activates a detecting device. Under the predicaments of quantum theory the system could be represented as a superposition of two configurations: in one the cat is alive, in the other the cat is dead. Observer's interference will actually determine which one of the two configurations will eventually collapse into a classical reality event.

accessible. Once the rational, computational mind and the state of consciousness focused on objective searching are dimmed and neutralized, then the inner, subjective VRT world returns to play its central role. The paralysis can be wiped off ("detersoque somno") and mental life reestablished. The process brings true substance to thought and it regenerates creativity.[5]

The myth concludes its message by describing how the rational mind, enlightened by the experience, now fully recognizes the centrality of the VRT realm in her own actualization, and its ultimate mystery. Once the stage is set by such recognition, the mind develops true and enduring affect linking and an enhanced ability for the full use of quantum consciousness. It achieves full possession of the vast knowledge ("totius orbis thesaurus") that resides in Eros' palace.

A myth is the ambiguous metaphor of a disguised knowledge: an enigma of sorts. While the main theme contains timeless substance, the interpretation of the intrinsic values, meaning, and content of the myth may undergo redefinition through time as our understanding of its inner message changes. After all, myths are the property of the myth's originators and of the myth's interpreters. No one really owns a myth's final and ultimate interpretation. As knowledge changes so does the meaning of the myth. It may be apt here to remember the words of Jonas Salk, "it will always be necessary to

---

[5]It may be interesting to reflect how the pregnancy state of Psyche seems to disappear, in the myth, with the disappearance of Eros. Psyche is just another of the virgins impregnated by gods who disseminate mythological history. But in her case the pregnant state seems to vanish once Eros has departed. Apuleius does not mention it any longer. Only at the end of the myth we are told that "thus in proper form Psyche was given in marriage to Eros. And when her time was come, a daughter was born to them, whom we call by the name Pleasure."

use metaphor and myth to provide 'comprehensible' guides to living. In this way, Man's imagination and intellect play vital roles in his survival and evolution" (1973, p. 82). The present revision of this particular myth is just another example. The theme is maintained; only some details are revised, as the interpretation of the metaphorical meaning of "Psyche" and "Eros." The myth's unfolding has just begun.

Conclusions

The subjective psychic equivalent of nonlocal coherence is briefly presented in the first vignette. Here, the subjective themes that dominated the self-disclosed material throughout the book reappear one final time, linked together in a vast simultaneous gestalt.

The vignette of Psyche and Eros documents the long history of human intuitive awareness that the individual mind is supported by collective universal knowledge and has ownership of this knowledge. It also proposes that this information exists in a form not accessible through rational, objective observation, but only by experiencing it into the subjective as a felt, presymbolic state. This state can be accessed through affectivity and is guided by laws different from the Newtonian ones.

CHAPTER TEN

Some Closing Reflections

"In the beginning God gave to every
people a cup of clay, and from this
cup they drank their life." Proverb of
the Digger Indians (Benedict, 1959,
p. xvi)

I have described in sequential way sets of events that
participate to the architectures of my mental operations. These architectures I have called gestalts. I experience these gestalts, however, not sequentially but in a
way that mystifies description: almost visually, as complex living holograms that contain a vast number of data
from events and states of affairs, which span through
time. The encounter with the gazelle carries a knowledge that emerged from the depths of the prehomi-
noideae evolutionary periods. The fire-making scenario
evokes images from the dawn of humanity. The shell
landscape taps into data from my ancestors' line. The
hat episode reveals a vast scenario of interconnected
personal experiential data that are unfolding from, and
are enfolded in, common affective attributes of an un-
conspicuous object. The tomato-slicing gestalt illustrates
how all the preceding data coexist in an interactive and
everchanging, rather immense mental configuration.

The events that constellate my subjective landscapes
have their specific real times in Newtonian reality.

Nonetheless, when the events coexist in a gestaltic field their real times appear to coexist too. (In other words, I am not aware of an "internal movie"; the internal time dimension, which would otherwise be a distinct element of my rational remembering, is missing under such VRT conditions.) This simultaneous coexistence contributes to ceaselessly updating the affectivity and intentionality of the gestalts. On the basis of my internal experience I can suggest that the product of such updating is contingent on where I am psychically at that specific moment, rather than representing a fixed algorithmic value. And it is an emergent structure, rather than a sum of its parts.[1]

I regularly experience all these gestaltic structures to be layered by a web of qualia states, as a diffuse energy field. Such energy field is not uniform among all states of affairs but creates or contributes to gradients of intensity that provide some of the perspective lines, of the dimensions directing VRT development. For some landscapes, such as the fire gestalt, affectivity is the prevailing dimension.

This last gestalt exemplifies for me a major problem in subjective research. It may be very difficult to reach intersubjective agreement on themes of genetic inheritance of complex webs of intentionality and affect-laden value systems. Figure 4.1 may help a bit: the images represent the expression (the collapse) of value systems and intentional networks enduring through speciations. Still, we may be eternally precluded from experiencing

---

[1]The *contingent* and the *emergent* attributes may explain why the entire temporal sequence needs to be always interactive in a timeless state, rather than being recalled each time as an already defined, calculated "sum" of past experiences to which the new one is "added."

with RT clarity motifs and mental states that are (have been) prevalently or exclusively nonverbal.[2]

Intersubjective confirmation will be a key element in the study of the subjective experience. We are vastly separated, different from each other, in the type of events and states of affairs that fill our mental landscapes. However, there is the possibility (or, as I prefer to think, the probability) that we share common thematic templates filled with differentiated elaborations of evolutionary knowledge.[3] I claim that we can therefore share the experiencing of such templates, whenever we restrain from casting blinding attentional light on individual components of the systems. Indeed, in order to experience the VRT working of the brain I need to achieve some dimming of rational thought. Only then do sections of the enchanted loom become more accessible to limited observation.[4]

Intersubjective exploration of what is "there" may represent the first step of the procedural ladder toward an understanding of subjectivity. We would then be able

---

[2]Eccles (1993) wrote, "I *feel* intensely that hominid evolution is the story of how I came to be. I can *sense* in my imagination the hazardous and tenuous evolutionary route pursued by remote ancestors in the millions of years of hominid evolution" (p. 239; emphasis added). I do not contend that in the fire gestalt I actually experienced a faint echo of "acting as a hominid," i.e., a consciousness of a formal hominid state within me. Rather, I experienced emotional states. These states, I contend, reflect stable and very old evolutionary programs. Adaptive achievements and options, such as bipedalism or the mastery of fire, have been hard to come by. It makes sense that they would be saved for future generations.

[3]As an aside, if one accepts my intuitive assessment of our mental content, one can see the futility of trying to compare a computer to a human mind. The silicon mind is a unidimensional fiction. Only a DNA-enriched computer could hope to acquire a section of the genetic library.

[4]I used my years of training in suspended listening and affect-linked free associational work to help me to master some ability in maintaining suspended attention and restrain from logical interference with the surfacing of VRT activity. I am therefore sufficiently comfortable in my *experiencing rather than reconstructing* these examples. Still, I realize the profound limitations attached to what I try to share.

to consensually validate the realm of the subjective, irrespective of the profound diversity in contents and in evolutionary variations that characterize the VRT world as compared to the neural level. To paraphrase Quine (1987, p. 133), looking at a shell fragment is the brutish neural event, which is replicable with significant stochastic accuracy, so that when you and I perform such action we are significantly more similar to than different from each other. Then there is the mentalistic (neuronal and subneuronal?) predicate of my subjective experience of "looking" at a shell fragment. This emergent mentalistic act of mine will be profoundly different from your "looking" at the same object, as chapter 6 made abundantly clear. The entire state of affairs from the combined neural and mentalistic functions represents my true and unreplicable reality on the issue of shell fragments.

Some critics may suggest that I imply lack of true ownership to our thoughts. My response is that we *brains* indeed think a lot, and very well, with marvelous depth. However, we may do most of our thinking before we translate our work into communicable schemata and "transmit" these schemata by means of our conscious self structure (a relational structure). All the knowledge exemplified in the preceding chapters—from antelopes and gorillas to tomatoes and Masters—seems to be instantaneously available, although in varying vastness, to the myriad of conscious operations that I perform during my daily existence. These conscious operations already represent an impressive feat of interconnected neural circuitry. The circuitry is further supported by the vast and always dynamically active field of "all-that-I-know."

When I engage in the process of making a decision I consider alternatives and consequences. These alternatives appear briefly at the periphery of my consciousness. They leave without residue, unnoticed, if they do not happen to activate a sequence related to the decision at issue. Or they may connect with the decision, and then evolve composite scenarios and outcomes that direct my choice of action.

After the action I may happen to say, "Oh! I did not consider (alternative X)." When I say that to myself I really mean either X did not show up or I did not see it within my consciousness field. Great planners evaluate an action against many alternatives (as Kasparov does) and have at their disposal a rich field of VRT information related to the action. Poor planners have a more barren field of alternatives, or lesser access to them. My point is that these alternatives do not originate in consciousness de novo, but are evoked into consciousness from another level, that of VRT activity. I also propose that the field in which genetic and epigenetic experiential knowledge is translated into adaptive images in a vast field of entangled quantum representations and probabilities that responds with complex collapses when influenced by some prevailing aspects of classical reality.

I am a brain. As a brain, I evolved intricate systems of adaptation (i.e., a mind), subject to continuous change, that have complex ontological underpinnings and complex developmental dynamics. These systems are organized into a "persona" or a self who is the expression of my (the brain's) negotiations with the environment in my ongoing quest for survival (security and satisfaction), and who appears to become an autonomous entity, a psychic reality separate from the physical reality of I-the-brain. Indeed, we-the-humans may be just a phase in the evolutionary expression of the brain. As humanity had to relinquish its centrality in the architecture of the planetary system and even more in that of the universe, so it may have to relinquish its centrality in the evolving adventure of the brain. In a nonlinear evolutionary universe—if it does exist—life will never get boring.

The sources of my functional adaptation can be traced, as can the sources of my structural adaptation, to the evolutionary requirements of life itself, to the evolutionary requirements of my own species, and to my personal evolutionary experiences. In the physical world, the site for the processing of such learning and of the intricate array of mental functions may involve the world of quantum mechanics as well as the world of classical physics. These concepts suggest that the architecture of the human mind may include sheer potentiality without actualization (the counterfactual mystery of quantum physics), profound subjectivity, unique and ultimately unreplicable ways of organizating experience. The brain may be the most complex object in the entire universe; *each one of us is "a most complex object in the entire Universe."* Therefore when we look at a human mind we look at something that we cannot see, but only infer about through empathy. This holds even more true in the case of distressed minds, where the flow of customary adaptive systems is under serious strain, and individual variance may become more prevalent.

Clearly, the introduction of the subjective into mental research will add profound complexity and instability to all attempts at understanding brain function. As I have tried to demonstrate we will be dealing with very large sets of data organized in configurations that will present significant variations among subjects and that will include elusive components as affectivity. The task of ordering this source of knowledge will indeed be formidable; but, so is the brain. Nature would not have turned to such an incredibly intricate organ for elaboration of data unless the data would indeed require it. I do not see any possibility of achieving true understanding of brain function until we begin to accept the existence and the importance of the subjective dimension and examine how we can in due time introduce this factor into the equation that may eventually describe the human mind.

It is befitting that I conclude with a final metaphor. During the most active planning of this book I frequently dreamed of oceans and became quite attracted by them. In one particular dream I was falling from a great height toward a majestic ocean of exquisite beauty, that was curving toward horizons of probabilistic, nebulous, almost nonexistent landmasses. I was falling into it as an observer in an experiment designed to study the ocean's ability to contain and dissolve concentrated waste matter. During the fall I felt no fear. I was actually sort of gliding down toward the water until I skidded on its surface and I found myself alone, on a small floating device. I did not sense any danger from its depth, but wonder and safety and intense gratification. I knew I could reach any distant shore I wanted, although my overt propelling ability was limited to my hands and feet. I am dimly aware that a sea of mental activity constantly moves within my mind and occasionally washes images ashore. This is my subjective world. Islands, even continents of visible self-structures emerge from the depths of my single, unified subjective ocean, whose waves keep redefining the lands of consciousness. The ocean contains local diversity in currents and depths and temperature ranges, but it is still *one* ocean, where all variations eventually transition into each other, all the time.

References

Apuleius (1989). *Apulei madavrensis metamorphoseon* (Liber 4, 5, 6). Cambridge, MA: Harvard University Press.

Asimov, I. (1991a). *Foundation edge*. New York: Bantam.

Asimov, I. (1991b). *Second foundation*. New York: Bantam.

Aspect, A., Grangier, P., & Roger, G. (1982). Experimental realization of Einstein-Podolsky-Rosen-Bohm *gedankenexperiment:* A new violation of Bell's inequalities. *Physics Review Letters, 46,* 91–94.

Benedict, R. (1959). *Patterns of culture*. New York: Mentor.

Bergman, I. (1956). *The seventh seal.* Videotape.

Bohm, D., & Hiley, B. J. (1993). *The undivided universe: An ontological interpretation of quantum theory*. New York: Routledge.

Borges, J. L. (1964a). Funes the memorius. In *Labyrinths: Selected stories and other writings* (pp. 59–66). New York: New Directions.

Borges, J. L. (1964b). The library of Babel. In *Labyrinths: Selected stories and other writings* (pp. 51–58). New York: New Directions.

Clissold, S. (Ed.). (1978). *The wisdom of St. Francis and his companions*. New York: New Directions.

Duane, D. (1986). The hand that feeds you. In *Thieves' world (Book 6): Wings of omen*. New York: Ace Fantasy.

Eccles, J. F. (1993). *Evolution of the brain: Creation of the self.* New York: Routledge.

Edelman, G. (1992). *Bright air, brilliant fire: On the matter of the mind*. New York: Basic Books.

Edelman, G. M. (1989). *The remembered present: A biological theory of consciousness*. New York: Basic Books.

Einstein, A., Podolsky, P., & Rosen, N. (1935). Can quantum-mechanical description of physical reality be considered complete? *Physics Review, 47,* 777–780.

Elsasser, W. M. (1969). A causal phenomena in physics and biology: A case for reconstruction. *American Scientist, 57,* 502–516.

Galin, D. (1994). The structure of awareness: Contemporary applications of William James' forgotten concept of "the fringe." *The Journal of Mind and Behavior, 15,* 375–401.

Galin, D. (1995). What is the difference between a duck? In J. Cohen & J. Schooler (Eds.), *Scientific approaches to consciousness: 25th Carnegie symposium on cognition, May 20–22, 1993* (pp. 1–7). Hillsdale, NJ: Erlbaum.

Galin, D. (1996). The structure of subjective experience: Sharpen the concept and terminology. In S. R. Hameroff, A. W. Kaszniak, & A. C. Scott (Eds.), *Toward a science of consciousness* (pp. 121–140). Cambridge, MA: MIT Press.

Gelernter, D. (1994). *The muse in the machine: Computerizing the poetry of human thought.* New York: Free Press.

Glanz, J. (1997). Mastering the nonlinear brain. *Science, 277,* 1758–1759.

Greenfield, S. A. (1995). *Journey to the centers of the mind: Toward a science of consciousness.* New York: W. H. Freeman.

Griffin, D. (1992). *Animal minds.* Chicago: University of Chicago Press.

Hameroff, S. R., Kaszniak, A. W., & Scott, A. C. (Eds.). (1996). *Toward a science of consciousness.* Cambridge, MA: MIT Press.

Hameroff, S. R., & Penrose, R. (1996). Orchestrated reduction of quantum coherence in brain microtubules: A model for consciousness. In S. R. Hameroff, A. W. Kaszniak, & A. C. Scott (Eds.), *Toward a science of consciousness* (pp. 507–540). Cambridge, MA: MIT Press.

Harman, W. H. (1996). Seeking an epistemology of subjectivity. In S. R. Hameroff, A. W. Kaszniak, & A. C. Scott (Eds.), *Toward a science of consciousness* (pp. 742–751). Cambridge, MA: MIT Press.

Hebb, D. O. (1949). *The organization of behavior.* New York: Wiley.

Herbert, N. (1993). *Elemental mind: Human consciousness and the new physics.* Penguin.

James, W. (1950). *Principles of psychology.* New York: Dover. (Original work published 1890).

Jung, C. G. (1968). The archetypes and the collective unconscious. In H. Read, M. Fordham, G. Adler, & W. McGuire (Eds.), In *The collected works of C. G. Jung* (Vol. 9). Princeton, NJ: Princeton University Press. (Original work published 1953).

Jung, C. G. (1977). Two essays on analytical psychology. In H. Read, M. Fordham, C. Adler, & W. McGuire (Eds.), *The collected works of C. G. Jung* (Vol. 7). Princeton, NJ: Princeton University Press. (Original work published 1953).

Kafatos, M., & Nadeau, R. (1990). *The conscious universe: Part and whole in modern physical theory.* New York: Springer-Verlag.

Kogan, N. (1980). *A cognitive style approach to metaphoric thinking.* Hillsdale, NJ: Erlbaum.

Lucretius (Titus Lucretius Carcus) (1992). *De rerum natura* (Liber 5). Cambridge, MA: Harvard University Press.

Mangan, B. (1991). *Meaning and structure of consciousness: An essay in psycho-aesthetics.* Doctoral dissertation, University of California, Berkeley. University Microfilms No. 920333636.

National Geographic Magazine (1996). *The urban gorilla.* Videotape.

Penrose, R. (1994). *Shadows of the mind: A search for the missing science of consciousness.* Oxford: Oxford University Press.

Plato (1973). *Phaedrus and the seventh and eighth letters.* Harmondsworth, U.K.: Penguin.

Quine, W. V. (1987). *Quiddities: An intermittent philosophical dictionary.* Cambridge, MA: Harvard University Press.

Salk, J. (1973). *Survival of the wisest.* New York: Harper & Row.

Schrodinger, E. (1980). The current state of affairs in quantum mechanics. *Proceedings of the American Physics Society, 124,* 323–338. (Original work published 1935).

Scott, A. C. (1995). *Stairway to the mind: The controversial new science of consciousness.* New York: Copernicus.

Searle, J. R. (1992). *The rediscovery of the mind.* Cambridge, MA: MIT Press.

Searle, J. R. (1993). *Intentionality: An essay in the philosophy of mind.* New York: Cambridge University Press.

Sherrington, C. S. (1951). *Man on his nature.* New York: Cambridge University Press.

Snell, B. (1986). *The discovery of the mind in Greek philosophy and literature.* New York: Dover. (Original work published 1896).

Sullivan, H. S. (1953). *The interpersonal theory of psychiatry.* New York: W. W. Norton.

Thuan, T. X. (1995). *The secret melody: And man created the universe.* New York: Oxford University Press.

Tuszynski, J. A., Trpisová, B., Sept, D., & Sataric, M. V. (1996). Microtubular self-organization and information processing capabilities. In S. R. Hameroff, A. W. Kaszniak, & A. C. Scott (Eds.), *Toward a science of consciousness* (pp. 407–418). Cambridge, MA: MIT Press.

Wallis Budge, E. A. (Ed., Trans.). (1960). *The Egyptian book of the dead.* Secaucus, NJ: University Books. (Original work published 1895).

Williams, N. (1997a). Evolutionary psychologists look for roots of cognition. *Science, 275,* 29–30.

Williams, N. (1997b). Selling Darwinism in a citadel of social science. *Science, 275,* 29.

Zohar, D. (1996). Consciousness and Bose-Einstein condensates. In S. R. Hameroff, A. W. Kaszniak, & A. C. Scott (Eds.), *Toward a science of consciousness* (pp. 439–450). Cambridge, MA: MIT Press.

Zoia, L. (1995). *Growth and guilt.* New York: Routledge.

Name Index

Apuleius, 154–155
Asimov, I., 14, 53
Aspect, A., 80n
Assisi, St. Francis, 69, 76–78

Benedict, R., 159
Bergman, I., 62
Bohm, D., 138, 139
Bomford, T., 84f
Borges, J. L., x, 92–93
Budge, W., 87

Clissold, S., 69, 76, 77–78
Cox, D. J., 84f
Cronin, H., 50n

Eccles, J. F., 15, 19–20, 135–136, 137n, 161n
Edelman, G. M., 15, 20–21, 38n, 58, 60, 109, 110, 118, 121, 122, 129, 132, 147
Einstein, A., 79–80, 139–140
Elsasser, W. M., 13

Frank, M., 149

Galin, D., xii–xiii, 6, 58n
Gelernter, D., 9, 15, 22–24, 55, 67, 75, 113, 123–124, 133
Glanz, J., 5
Grangier, P., 80n
Greenfield, S. A., 15, 21–22, 58, 135–136
Griffin, D., 74

Hameroff, S. R., 137, 140
Harman, W. H., 6, 15, 26–27

Hauser, M., 50n
Hebb, D. O., 38n
Herbert, J., 15
Herbert, N., 17–18, 19, 41n, 118, 138–139
Herodotus, 105–106n
Hiley, B. M., 138, 139
Hollis, J., 92

James, W., xii, 27–28n, 34, 58n
Jung, C. G., 1, 91–92, 103

Kafatos, M., 138
Kasparov, G., 61, 62–65, 66, 67n
Kaszniak, A. W., 140
Kogan, N., 9

Lanting, F., 84f
Lucretius, 47

Mangan, B., 58n

Nadeau, R., 138

Pelorat, J., 53
Penrose, R., 15, 20, 66n, 80n, 135, 137, 140
Pinker, S., 50n
Plato, 31
Podolsky, P., 79–80

Quine, W. V., 162

Roger, G., 80n
Rosen, N., 79–80

Salk, J., 157–158

171

Sanguineti, V., ix
Sataric, M. V., 137
Schrodinger, E., 79–80, 156
Scott, A. C., 5, 8n, 13, 15, 25–26,
     27–28n, 117, 135–136, 140
Searle, J. R., 7, 18, 41–42, 62, 80,
     124–125, 126n
Sept, D., 137
Sherrington, C. S., 8
Snell, B., 106n
Sullivan, H. S., 119

Thuan, T. X., 121n
Trpisová, B., 137
Tuszynski, J. A., 137

Voltaire, 150n

Williams, N., 50n

Zohar, D., 136, 140n
Zoia, L., 105–106n

Subject Index

Acculturation, Greek process of, 105–106n
Adaptation
data for, 16
evolutionary, xv
functional, 164
Adaptive knowledge, 38–39
Adaptive programs, inherited, 50
Affect, 41. See also Affectivity;
Emotional states;
Emotions; Feeling;
Feeling states
high and low focus states in, 22–25
in inherited knowledge, 51
Affect linking, 23, 28
attention in, 60
with element of fire, 89–90
healing quality of, 131–132
to values, 113–116
Affect-based system, 15
Affective connectedness, 117–133
Affective loading, 16
Affective recognition, 95–96
Affective resonance, xvi
Affective weighting, 141–143
Affectivity, xvi, 118–121, 155. See also Affect
of gestalts, 160
liability of, 67n
in memory recovery and linkage, 24–25
in perceptual recategorization, 141
rational mind and, 156–157
African social gestalts, 109
Agamemnon, 105n
Aloneness, 70

Alternate personalities, ix–xii
Ambiguity, 141–143, 147–148
Ambiguous mental states, 9–11
Ancestors' lines, xv, 44–45, 51
values from, 103–112, 115
Anthropic principle, 121
Anthropomorphizing, 78–80
Archetypal world, 44n
Archetypes, 91–92, 103
ancestral line-specific, 105–108
evolutionary, 87–101
Artificial intelligence, high-focus thought in, 22–23
Aspectual shape, 42
Attention
in affect linking, 60
dimming of, 60
focus levels of, 22–25, 55–56, 68, 133
in mental focus, 68
suspended, 161n
Awareness, two parts of, xiin

Background, 42
Behavioral adaptation, 50
Brain
connectedness of, 13–14
quantum activity in, 19–20
reptilian, 93
Brain-mind complex, xiii–xiv. See also Mental functioning; Mind

Causality, 26
Cerebral functioning, global, 4–5
Chess
Kasparov-Deep Blue match, 61–67

as mathematical game, 62–63
Collective unconscious, 103
  conscious recognition of,
    112–115, 116
  cultural values and, 103–112,
    115
Communication, interspecies,
  69–86
Communicative devices, 59–60
Communion, 70, 71–73
Computational power, 62–63
  attention and, 68
  subjectivity and, 135–136
Computer mind, 161n
Concentric consciousness
  theory, 21–22
Connectedness, 49–50, 111
  affective, 117–133
  mythical, 92
  to nature, 73–86
  primeval, 82–83
  secure, 88–89
  universal, 143–146, 148
Consciousness
  cosmic, undivided, 138–139
  data contributing to, 68
  definition of, 58
  fear of, 7
  focused attention level of,
    22–25, 55–56, 68, 133
  hierarchies of, 25–27
  higher-order, 60, 147
  I-am-a-brain level of, 163–164
  selfhood and, 60–61
  structural levels of, 59n
  subjective element of, xii–xiii
  two orders of, 137–138,
    146–147
  unconscious thinking and, xiv,
    36–37, 53–68
Cosmic religious feeling, 139–140
Countertransference
  phenomena, 14

Creation, communion with,
  46–47
Creativity, 9
  unstructured thinking and,
    123–124
  very rapid thought and,
    156–157
Cultural archetypes, Western,
  104–105
Cultural niches, xv
Cultural values, 103–112, 115
Curiosity, xv

Darwinian theory, 95
Deep Blue, 61–67
Derivative adaptation, 39
Design bias, 8–9
Developmental themes, 43–49
Diffuse attention state, 23–24
Divergent thinking, 9
Divine retribution, 105
DNA, junk, 82–83
Dominance behavior, 84
Dynamic adaptation, 39

Emotional halo, 122–123
Emotional recognition, xv
Emotional states
  evolutionary sharing of, 78–86
  presemantic, 90–91
Emotions. *See also* Affect;
    Affectivity; Emotional
    states; Feeling; Feeling
    states
  definition of, 41
  labeling of, 119
Empathy, xv
Enchanted loom, 8
Epistemology, characteristics of,
  26–27
Eros myth, 153–158
Evolution
  adaptations of, xv

sequence of, 110
Evolutionary archetypes, 87–101
Evolutionary knowledge, loss of, 99, 101
Evolutionary sharing, 78–86
Experience, xv. *See also*
Subjective experience
Experiential learning
developmental themes in, 43–49
exponential increase in, 40
versus inherited knowledge, 109–111
Exploration process, 26
External reality, subjective view of, 117–118

Fairytales, 91
Familiarity-recognition-connectedness complex, 105–107, 111, 112, 115–116, 131, 135, 147
quantum coherence and, 139
Feeling. *See also* Affect; Affectivity; Emotional states; Emotions; Feeling states
definition of, 118
sea of, 119
undefined, 119
units of. *See* Qualia
Feeling states, clarifying role of, 40–41
Feeling structures, 123–124
Felt attributes, interactive reality, 126–128, 133
Fire
affect linking with, 89–90
taming of, 89, 92–93, 100
Focused attentional states, 22–25, 55–56, 68, 133
emotions and, 123–124

Genetic drives, 120

Genetic endowment, 37–39, 85–86
junk DNA and, 82–83
objective example of, 76–85
personal example of, 69–76
recognition of, 73–76
Genetic intelligence, 37–39
creating commonality, 50
Genetic library, 92–93
vestigial functions in, 93–95
Gestalt consciousness, 21–22
Gestaltic structures, 159–160
Gestaltic view, 15
Gestalt(s), 32, 159
cultural, 106–107
fire-setting, 87–91
formation of, 150–152
sensory, 142
simultaneous coexistence of, 135, 147
social, 105–109
structural neuronal, 22
subjective, 4–5, 128–130
vastness of, xvi
very rapid thinking, 125–126
Global data elaboration, nonconscious, 24–25
Godel's theorem, 66*n*
Gorillas, intentionality in, 78–82
Grand Illusion, 118
Greek hero, 105*n*
Group togetherness, 88–89
Guernica, subjective perception of, 12–13

Habituation process, 142
Hero concept, 105
Hidden words, 75
Hierarchical system, 15, 25–27
Hominid evolution, 89, 161*n*
common knowledge of, 50
Hominoideae
evolution of, 50, 89, 161*n*

legacy of, 95
Hubris, 105

Idiosyncratic development, 43–49
Iliad, 105n
Illusion, 142–143
Immense numbers, 13
Indeterminism, xiv
Individual experiential learning,
　40
Individualized decisions, 37–38,
　40
Inherited adaptive style, 50
Inherited knowledge, xiv–xv, 111
　versus experiential learning,
　　109–111
　intentionality and affect in, 51
　layers of, 38–39, 50
Instincts, 37, 120
Intelligence, genetic, 37–39, 50
Intelligence tests, design bias of, 9
Intentional states, intertwined,
　41–42
Intentionality, 32–33, 41–42,
　124–126, 133
　in computational science, 135
　of gestalts, 160
　in inanimate objects, 130–131
　in inherited knowledge, 51
　nonconscious, 125
　refined webs of, 120
Interactive reality, 121–124,
　132–133
　characterizing, 133
　intentionality in, 124–126
Internal objects
　subjective experience of,
　　126–129
　validity and importance of,
　　122–123
Interspecies communication,
　69–86
Intersubjective validation, 58n

Intrauterine development, 93n
Intrinsic value systems, 39–40
Introspective method, 32
Intuition, 16, 56–57, 137–138,
　147, 155
　in chess, 64–65
　a component of intelligence, 9
　in mental processes, 65–66
I-the-brain, 137, 146–147,
　163–164
I-the-self, 137
I-the-self consciousness, 147

Ka, 94
Kasparov-Deep Blue chess
　match, 61–67
Knowledge
　data contributing to, xiv–xv
　disguised, 157–158
　experiential, 162–163
　hierarchies of, 25–27
　inherited, xiv–xv, 38–39, 50,
　　51, 109–111
　interconnectivity of, 28, 33

Language, limitation of, 31
Learning, known sources of, 32
Life
　energy of, 119
　unfolding of, 69–86
Linear mathematics, 5

Master, search for, 96–99
Meaning, 120
　"sameness of," 106–107
Memories-images, 90
Mental activity, xvi
　quantum mechanics of,
　　135–136
Mental evolution, adaptive
　changes in, 100
Mental functioning

consciousness and unconscious
in, 53–68
feeling aspect of, 133
models of, 15–16
objective observations of,
27–28
quantum mechanics and, 22, 43
sequence of, 140–141
subjective gestalts in, 4–5
unity of, 19
Mental leaps, 23
Mental objects
definition of, 117
felt qualities of. *See* Qualia
Mental phenomena, 7–8
Mental research
on affect and thought, 22–25
concentric consciousness
theory in, 21–22
on hierarchical systems, 25–27
neuronal group selection
theory in, 20–21
on quantum consciousness,
17–20
subjectivity and, 6–27
Mental self, development of, xiii
Mental states
ambiguous, 9–11
high and low focus, 22–25
intentionality in, 124–126
interconnected, 150–152
subjectivity and, 6–7
Mental systems
complexity of, 13–14
immense number of, 13
Mental units, 137*n*
Mentalistic portraits, 31–52
Mind
social, 120
Mind(s). *See also* Brain; Mental
activity; Mental
functioning; Mental states
architecture of, 164

conscious and unconscious
workings of, 53–68
diversity of, 28–29
"Einsteinian" architecture of,
129
as gestalt, xiii–xiv
map of, 16
social, 120
Mood, 119
Motus animi, 41
Myth, 91, 157–158

Nature
communion with, 46–47, 70,
71–73
uncontrollable, 92
Necker cube, 9–11
Needs, 120
evolution of, 95
feeling structures and, 88–89
intrinsic and acquired, 39–40
primitive, xv
Nemesis, 105
Network, intentional, 42
Neural circuitry
interconnected, 162–163
quantum mechanics of,
136–137
stimulus perception and
recognition in, 2–3
Neural Darwinism, 15, 20–21
Neural recognition systems, 110
Neuronal assemblies, 38
Neuronal group selection
theory, 20–21
Neurons
cytoskeleton of, 137
quantum events in, 20
Newtonian laws, quantum
randomness and, 17–18
Newtonian mechanics, xiii–xiv
Newtonian physics, 136, 147,
159–160

Nonconscious intentionality, 125
Nonconscious process, 68
Nonconscious work, 59–60
Nonlinear systems, 5
Nonlinearity, 25–26
    dynamics of, 16
Nonlocal coherence, 138–139,
    147
Nonlocality principle, 80n
Numinosity experience, 77,
    111–112, 115–116, 135,
    139–140, 147
    in experience of fireplace,
    89–90

Objective studies
    bias of design in, 8–9
    limitations of, 27–28
    reductionistic, 7–8, 13–14, 29
Observed reality, 18–19
Observer effect, 8
Odyssey, 105–106n
ORC gene, 93n
Origin-recognition-complex
    proteins, 93–94

Paleosymbols, 95
Paradox mystery, 97
Paranoia, 99
Perception
    ambiguity in, 141–143
    subjectivity of, 11–13
    veridical, 129
Perception-response, objective
    studies of, 7–8
Perceptual bootstrap, 110, 121
Perceptual categorization, 121,
    125
    affectivity and, 141
    of interactive reality, 133
    of object attributes, 127–129
Persona, 163
Personal experience, selection
    process for, 33–34

Personal inclinations, 3–4
Personal vignette, 53–61
Phylogenetically ancient roots, 82
Pietá, subjective perception of,
    12–13
Preprogrammed behavioral
    responses, 37
Presynaptic system, 13–14
Presynaptic vesicular grid, 19–20
Primal human evolution, xv
Primary repertoire, 20–21
Primeval experiencing, 82–83
Primordial types, 91–92
Progeny survival, 119–120
Prometheus myth, 100
Protohuman programs, 96–98,
    100–101
Psyche
    myth of, 153–158
    subjective study of, 14
Psychic entities, everlasting, 94
Psychic reality, 163–164
Psychic structures, 118–119
    feeling attributes of, 120
Psychons, 137

Qualia, 32, 120, 132
    definition of, 41, 117
    in mental events, 137
    sharing of, 74
    sources of, 118–119
    web of, 117–133, 160
Quanta, 132
    web of, 135–148
Quantum coherence, 138–139
Quantum consciousness
    theories, 15
Quantum indeterminacy, 17–18
Quantum inseparability, 19–20
Quantum mechanics
    in mental events, 135–136
    in mental function, 22, 43
Quantum physics, 136

versus Newtonian physics, 147
Quantum randomness, 17–18
Quantum systems, 138
  entangled, 138–141
Quantum theory, xiii–xiv
  mystery of, 80n
Quantum thinglessness, 18–19
Quantum wave, 137–138

Racial knowledge, 50
Rational mind, 154–155
  affectivity and, 156–157
Rational thinking, high-focus,
  123–124
Reality
  ambiguous, 141–143, 147–148
  classical, 147
  infinite centers of, 129
  interactive, 121–126, 132–133
  Newtonian, 159–160
  objective versus subjective, 141
  psychic, 163–164
  recategorization of, 144–146
  subjective perception of,
    ix–xiii, 11–13, 165–166
  value-driven categorization of,
    147–148
Reductionistic replicable
  approach, 29
Reentry process, 21
Relational structure, 162
Relational thinking, 33–34, 37,
  59, 68, 109
  ideas expressed in, 155
Relaxed mental state, 23
Remembered present, 58
Replicability argument, 8–9
Representational constructs, 16
Reptilian brain, 93
Rightness, feelings of, 58n

Satisfaction
  definition of, 119

as driving force, 132
  intentionality and, 125–126
  qualia and, 120
Schroder stairs, 9–11
Schrodinger's cat, 97
Schrodinger's creatures, 156n
Secondary repertoire, 21
Security, 88–89
  definition of, 119–120
  as driving force, 132
  intentionality and, 125
  qualia and, 120
Self, representational constructs
  and, 16
Self-disclosure
  avoidance of, xii–xiii
  process of, 32–33
Selfhood, 27
  conscious and unconscious
    mind in, 60–61
  consciousness and, 58
  enduring state of, 152–153
  personal history of, 44–49, 51
  subjectivity and, 35–36
Self-images, 61n
Semantic bootstrapping, 109, 110
Sensory gestalt, 142
Social gestalts
  African, 109
  Western, 105–109
Social mind, 120
Sociocultural adaptation, 39
Sociocultural knowledge, 50
Space theme, 70
Spirituality, in diffuse attention
  states, 24
Stillness, 70, 72
Stimulus, perception and
  recognition of, 2–3
Structural neuronal gestalts, 22
Subjective essence, 117–118
  affectivity and, 118–121
Subjective experience

in computational science,
    135–136
definition of, 117–118
intersubjective confirmation
    of, 161–162
in mental function, 65–66
overview of, 1–29
reluctance to reveal, xii–xiii
Subjective filter, 120–121
Subjective gestalt, 4–5, 128–129
    behavioral outcomes of,
        129–130
Subjective reality, 11–13, 165–166
    uncertainty of, ix–xiii
Subjective self, casual approach
    to, 34–35
Subjective studies, 11–13
Subjectivity, 28
    centrality of, 6–7
    definition of, 1–6
    mental research and, 6–27
    scarcity of data on, 31–32
    versus science, xi–xii
    selfhood and, 35–36
Subneuronal system, 13–14
Survival needs
    assessment of, 146–147
    subjective experience centered
        on, 131–132
Suspended attention, 161n
Symbolic thought, 137
Synaptic metastability, 38n

Territorial programs, 84
Territorial themes, 70
Territoriality, xv, 39–40
Thinking affectivity, directed
    versus undirected,
    123–124
Thought. *See also* Rational
    thinking; Relational
    thinking; Very rapid
    thinking state

creative, 123–124, 156–157
high and low focus states in,
    22–25, 133
Topobiological competition,
    20–21

Unconscious
    consciousness and, 36–37
    focused attention level and,
        55–56
    selfhood and, 60–61
The Undivided Universe, 139
Unexpected connections, 23
Unity of experience, 26
Universal connectedness,
    143–146, 148
Universe, space-time fabric of,
    138–139

Value systems, 39–40
    acquired, 39–40
    affective linking and, 113–116
    expression of, 160
    time reworking, 104–105
Values, 120
    from collective unconscious,
        103–112, 115
    evolution of, 87–101
    nonshifting, 96–97
    primitive, xv
Vast intentional web, 125–126
Very rapid thinking, 16, 25,
    33–34, 68, 135, 160
    attention dimming and, 60
    certainty about, 114–115
    collapse of, 123
    creativity and, 156–157
    familiarity-recognition-
        connectedness feeling
        in, 139
    information from, 163
    intuitive certainty about, 106
    I-the-brain consciousness in,
        146–147

states of, 58–59
unconscious, 37
Vast network of, 125–126,
 137–138
Vestigial functions, 93–94
Vestigial structures, $93n$

Wave of possibilities, 17–18

Weighting phenomenon,
 141–143
Western culture
 archetypes of, 104–105
 Greek roots of, $106n$
Wild animals, communicating
 with, 73–86
Words, transparent, 98–99